PAUL BURKE'S
NEO-DIETER'S HANDBOOK

WHEN WE LOST OUR NUTRITIONAL ROOTS;
WHERE TO FIND THESE FOODS TODAY

- *LOSE FAT*
- *GAIN MUSCLE*
- *HELP HEAL CHRONIC ILLNESS*
- LIVE LONGER
- *REDUCE INFLAMMATION*
- *SLOW AGING*

PAUL T. BURKE

ISBN: 1-4392-4541-X
ISBN-13: 9781439245415
Library of Congress Control Number: 2009908173

Visit www.booksurge.com to order additional copies.

Note for Librarians: A cataloguing record for this book is available
from Library and Archives United States at

DEDICATION

As always, there are many people—writers, scientists, and other professionals—who have touched my life during the course of studying about this topic and writing this book, which I believe is of historical, present-day, and future value. To all of those whose work I have read, I thank you for all of the painstaking time which you have each invested in your works. This enables others, such as myself, to stand on your shoulders and reach ever higher to the gateway of each mind on this planet that we call Earth. To the anthropologists and archeologists who spend their entire lives unearthing and studying the bones, diets, icons, deities, cultural artifacts, and the many other thousands of pieces our ancestral puzzle, I thank you from the bottom of my heart. Without all of your work and enormous efforts, this book couldn't have been written.

As a boy, I used to dig up antique bottles from the eighteenth and nineteenth centuries, and I got a firsthand thrill from discovering what a mother drank, what food was fed to her first child, whether there was dysentery in the family, and whether they drank "bitters" or whiskey. I got to dig through three or four centuries of earth that revealed everything from brown "barrel" bitters bottles, to rectangular dysentery cork-tops, to a flask with our first president on one side and the great American general Zachary Taylor on the other—that was the find of a lifetime. As a young man, I saw the meaning and value of recreating the past and imagining what it must have been like for dozens and then hundreds of lonely outcasts—from England, France, and other countries—to make it across the Atlantic Ocean, to piece together a log home, and to make peace and war with the aboriginals of North America. By finding such bottles while digging through the ancient soil, I could hear the voices of our country's earliest settlers and their friends and foes alike. I can only imagine the feeling of stumbling upon the ancient cave drawings and paintings of Lascaux (France) or unearthing "Lucy" (our first "mother"), discovered in 1974 by anthropologist Professor Donald Johanson and his student Tom Gray in a maze of ravines at Hadar in northern Ethiopia. These are greater clues as to who we are, what we did, and where we came from.

Although this is a book about nutrition, I also draw on what I have learned from others, from my daily trips to the Natural History Museum in New York City, and from reading hundreds of books on mythologies and aboriginal cultures—what they ate and their way of life. From all of these sources, I drew my own conclusions about our evolutionary past, and it is my intention to spread this knowledge and wisdom in order to help all who read it. In addition, as we read about our historical nutrition and review our present nutrition, we have but one question: from whence does the future come? The answer lies amongst these pages going forward, remembering always those who have passionately searched the ancient world, beneath the enormity in stages of soils of eons of time, for clues to inform all of us of the answers of today and tomorrow, for no greater statement has ever been made than, "*The future lie sleeping beneath the blankets of our past.*" For that, I thank all of those who have awoken the past in order for many to see the future.

———

ACKNOWLEDGEMENTS

It is not a secret that my intellectual mentor was Professor Chandler Steiner, formerly a professor of philosophy at Cambridge College, and a PhD of philosophy and theology from Cambridge University in England. I have written about him in many of my published writings, books, and articles, for he was a brilliant man who constantly probed my mind and my soul for more than I thought that I could ever tolerate, while I uncovered more about the world than I ever knew was possible. He brought me from the eccentric life that I had led and told me how to use that eccentricity for the good of my life, for the good of all with whom I came into contact.

He left us all too soon, for he was a true genius with the inquisitiveness and the personality of Socrates himself—Chandler's first teacher-model. Without Chandler having taught me how to ask the unusual questions and grind the hatchet against the stone in such a way as to form a double edge (the metaphor for all life on this earth), then I would not have been able to complete the books that I have written. Questioning the present paradigm of eating is no different to me than questioning why one muscle on my body grew so easily and another gave me so much trouble. His whisper is always in my ear when I write. I hope you hear him in some of my words.

It has been said that "*no man is an island*" and "*behind every great man stands a woman*." I would say that Karin, my passionate partner in life, understands these two appropriate—if not ancient—idioms, perhaps better than most. Karin really stands beside me in every way and ahead of me in ways that I never saw anyone do before. Yet her true spirit behind her tender words is always encouragement. Although she looks at least a decade younger than her true age, Karin has wisdom beyond her years; however, she too has had some of her own dilemmas regarding this culture's perspective about eating. In fact, this book would not have been written had it not been for her belief in me and what I have learned about our ancient ancestors, what they ate, and why. As with so many women, she prides herself on taking care of her body, and that accounts for her youthful appearance; as I stated previously, however, her wisdom is beyond her years, and my love for her grows daily. A true entrepreneurial spirit, she lifts me up when the sun dies down, and she brings me to earth if my eagerness to teach the world strays off course. She has brought me great love and joy. For me to see her each day is a blessing that I never thought that I would glimpse.

Bill Koch is well known in certain circles, and many of you may be familiar with some of his greatest achievements (winning the America's Cup and forming the first all-women team to defend the Cup). Regardless of what you may have heard or read about Bill, he is a man with a heart as big as his houses and yachts, and with an intellect to create such things personally. He is a "hands-on" kind of guy, and he continues to inspire me as he quietly runs one of the world's most powerful companies.

———

TABLE OF CONTENTS

PREFACE

If ever there were a time and a place to read about the how, what, where, and why of human nutrition, it is now. No greater challenge lies ahead for Americans than our health care management and the future of our food supply. After decades of doctors and many other professionals denying the link between what one chooses to eat and one's health, finally, the once small bubble has burst. Even those who once breathed fire against "holistic healing," "whole foods," and "health nuts" are all now presented with the results of scientific trials, medical journal writings, and many doctors alike agreeing that what one eats does make a difference in one's health.

Yet in no other time in our history has there been so many young type I and type II diabetics as there are today. At no other time in history has there been such an abundance of food that people actually eat it and then vomit it for fear of becoming obese. It is astonishing what the icons of the culture portray as reality, and what many women (and men) are willing to do to look like those figurine iconoclastic beings. Food, in a word, has become "dangerous" in many ways.

The underlying reasons for which I wrote this book are threefold. First, I have a genuine belief that the human mind can not only become intellectually brilliant, but can also become disciplined in daily rituals. This discipline is needed in order to discard the scourge of processed foods and rely on what I believe is the everlasting nutritional program of all humans since the dawn of our existence as thinking, hunting, and gathering Upper-Paleolithic, Paleolithic, and Neolithic beings.

Secondly, there seems to be a need to rethink what we are doing in our culture in the sense that everyone is in a hurry, which often leads to poor choices and life-threatening mistakes when eating. I always ask, "*In a hurry to do what? In a hurry to go where?*" This hectic pace is what causes so many to grab a pizza to go, or a steak and cheese hoagie to eat while driving. I have always wondered why someone would purposefully poison his or her body just to get someplace two minutes sooner or to make an extra hundred bucks. I also have always been baffled by people who say to me, "*You don't eat ice cream? Or donuts? You must feel as though you live in a prison!*" No, it is those who are addicted to certain foods who are imprisoned; they will be chained to the health-care system before long—if they are not already—and forever chained they will stay. How hard is it to make a good, healthy lunch to bring to work each day? For most, it is much harder than it is to eat processed junk food on the run and then end up going to the doctor with the hope of a "cure" by way of a pill.

Lastly, I feel that I have lived the life that I do in order to give something back to those who may not know or who may not sit down to contemplate what they are eating (and doing) and why. I have been blessed with both the greatest of highs and the most tragic of lows. The highs have ranged from winning major bodybuilding and arm-wrestling championships to having principal roles in movies. I have also had a long, prosperous, and wonderful career as a trainer to everyone from famous celebrities to Bill Koch's winning America's Cup team. One of the lows is that I have battled multiple sclerosis now for fifteen years. Every neurologist whom I ever saw told me, while looking at the two ominous and obvious lesions in my spinal cord (at C-2 and C-4) on MRI film, that eventually I would be confined to a wheelchair as a quadriplegic because of the size and location of these lesions. Today, fifteen years after diagnosis, I am six feet tall and weigh 220 pounds of rock-hard muscle. I can leg press 800 pounds ten times, and I can bench press over 315 pounds for eight repetitions. I can kick-box, arm wrestle, and do anything that one can imagine a lifelong bodybuilder and lover of pugilism (i.e., boxing) could do. How did I stop the scourge of MS? By eating the way I describe in this book and by modifying my exercise routines to give my body more rest. I have studied our entire evolution— from chimpanzee, to hominoid, to *Homo sapiens*, to modern day "*Techno sapiens*," and all the eras that fall in between. The human body has come a long way. The human mind has yet to peak, and this is what fascinates me about the humans of today— their choices in both nutrition and exercise. I have written about and published both topics, but I felt it was time to really express all of my deepest thoughts and knowledge about the modern-day nutritional dilemma which we face in our culture.

I have experienced some tremendously rewarding moments as an athlete. I won my share of arm-wrestling contests in the U.S. and Europe, stood on center stage a number of times as the winner of bodybuilding championships, sailed with the America's Cup team, and had speaking roles in famous TV shows (*Spenser for Hire*) and movies (*Mystic Pizza*). I also played my childhood idol, Steve Reeves, as "Hercules," in an internationally shown Wendy's commercial. I have rubbed elbows with some of the biggest names in show business and financial business, and I have trained and befriended many of them during that process. The point is that I have seen life from many vantage points. I grew up poor and under the tyranny of alcoholism. I was in a traveling carnival and circus by the age of sixteen, and I made that huge leap of faith to join the U.S. Air Force at nineteen years old. While in the Air Force, I was the first airman overseas to win a bodybuilding contest, and I became a European arm-wrestling champion for three years. I gave many motivational speeches to the U.S. Air Force Recruiters Conventions and to Air Force personnel in USAFE (United States Air Force Europe). These speeches were all designed to educate and share my knowledge with those who gave me so much. The military changed my life. I began with a life of running away from alcoholism and abuse, followed by entering the weird and wacky world of being a carnie— making the decision to enter the military opened the world up to me. It offered me a place to begin what would become my love, my passion, and my dream—the exercise and study of the human body.

Something tells me that many of you think that there is a magic bullet to living life to its fullest, to getting into shape, to losing those last few inches around your waist or thighs, or to recovering from a chronic illness—I'm here to tell you that there is no magic bullet. However, there is knowledge and wisdom to guide you; as with all of my books and writings, I am going to share it all with you, from the abundance of my heart, soul, and passion—all that I know and use myself. Within the pages of this book, you will discover the missing link which is absent from so many diets out there in a wasteland of confusion surrounding what we should be eating and why. There are so many quick fixes, and they are just that—quickly adopted ideas, and just as quickly discarded delusions.

You will also find yourself understanding, perhaps for the first time, why you may not be able to embrace life, conquer your fears, and seize what is rightfully yours. So much of what we eat changes our moods, our ability to be creative, and our ability to thrive, live, and love vibrantly. You owe it to yourself and to your children to read this book, contemplate it, and use your natural, intrinsic logic to understand that there can only be one truly human way to eat. This is not a book of smoke and mirrors, nor of gimmickry; it is instead a reflection on the past in order to understand our ancestral heritage, our present, and our future. You have control over much more than you may believe. So come… come with me now on a short, but wisdom-laden journey—a journey, as has been said before, back to the future.

———

INTRODUCTION

I have been studying about the human body all of my life, whether in academia or on my own. I started bodybuilding at age twelve (and continue to train at fifty-three years old), and I started reading about historical and contemporary nutrition at age eighteen (and continue to do so). Nothing has kept me busier or more focused than working with the magnificent, fascinating, scientific, biomechanical, mystical, and mesmerizingly infinite human body.

From all that studying and questioning, I have written over five hundred peer-reviewed published articles, published two books (with two more on the burner), and trained over two thousand athletes, celebrities, and business professionals, both men and women. Through it all, I have seen and witnessed some really amazing results and observed strange medical anomalies changed by mere dietary compromises. I have helped those who have had everything from bulimia and anorexia, to multiple sclerosis and rheumatoid arthritis. I have yet to meet a person who does not immediately lose fat, gain muscle, feel better, look younger, and feel less depressed and more able to focus once on the diet that I am about to reveal to you in this book. Before I do this, I want to tell you how I came to the conclusions that are presented in this book.

The one common thread that seems so apparent to me is that women in our culture worry about "gaining weight." They also begin to do such things as induce vomiting after eating, binge after a strict diet, and stop eating altogether—those are the problems that I see most often. There are many other stories that we all know and have heard related. These behaviors are not only damaging to the body - they are not necessary; there is a more natural way to prevent weight gain.

On the other hand, I see men injecting themselves with human growth hormone (HGH), taking anabolic steroids, and taking many, many nonessential food supplements to get "*bigger muscles and six-pack abs.*" Again, these results can be obtained without the unnecessary dangers that can accompany the abuse of steroids and HGH.

Here is the truth: there is a way to eat that will cure all of these ills in our culture, whether you want to lose or to gain weight. This way of eating which I am revealing here is really a miracle in the sense that we developed, evolved, and stopped organically evolving under very specific nutritional factors and elements. It is what we ate when our evolutionary bodies stopped organically evolving that matters most, and this way of eating has been written about in many anthropological texts and is even mentioned in tablets dating back 7,500 years ago. Some have even gone so far as to believe that this way of eating—which changed so drastically during a very critical time in our evolution—is the historical and Biblical symbol for the "*fall of man*." (This is said to be symbolic in the sense that pre-agrarian man was a hunter-gatherer— close to, and an integral part of, nature. Once those ways were changed to plant and animal domestication—dominating nature and extracting man from nature—the very essence of being human changed. We "fell" into an abyss.) That essence of what is poetic, what is mythological, and what is real, is so critical to understand in order to allow us to move forward with the way that our eating has evolved—certainly not what we ate after this hunter-gatherer period, and most important of all, *not* what we are eating today as a society.

We all grow up believing that what we eat must be good for us because our parents said so. We watch and mimic what our parents eat (ate), and as their children, we then pass down our experiences with food to our children (except for me and my children, and hopefully you and yours). However, most children in the United States are fed far too much sugar and refined food (what I have called "faux-food"). However, it does go deeper than this; just think of the savage beating your cells take from eating that junk as a child! That sets you up for a tough time later in life.

As children, we had (and today's kids still have) virtually nothing upon which to base an argument against what our parents taught us, and in this new millennium - for sure this new century - children are being fed the absolute worst foods imaginable. Of course, being children, they show few overt symptoms other than bouncing off the living room walls after ice cream and brownies, and crashing an hour later, slumped over their car seats. Then we assume they must need a drug—so goes the way of the culture.

Thus, we also believed as children—since our bodies rarely seemed to have any overt, correlative negative effects from what we ate—that even the mounds of candy, chocolate, and ice cream that we consumed as children had no negative effects on our bodily health. How wrong that turns out to be.

We also assumed that our school systems gave us food that must have been good for us, for why would they do otherwise? They all based their decisions on what was considered healthy by the Food and Drug Administration (FDA) and the required daily allowance (RDA) charts (which mysteriously change every decade). Our parents also watched advertisements on the three network TV stations which were the only stations around; perhaps more importantly, they believed what doctors had told them (through charts and other visual aids), that food had little to no consequences on our young, but developing bodies. When Ronald Reagan was president, he once said that ketchup is a vegetable. Really? How can that be? Nothing which humans have made is a "real food."

The following is an article that I wrote over a decade ago about the subject of children, nutrition, aging, and energy.

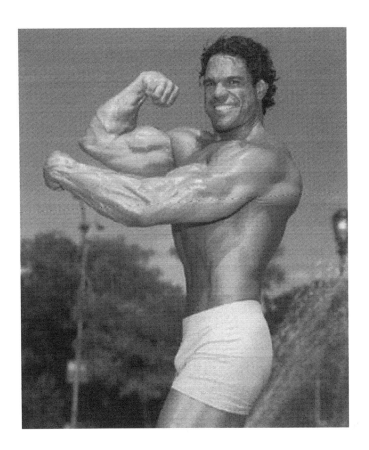

F Since I live in New York City, I usually prefer walking to the gym on my workout days rather than taking a cab or subway. This allows me to build another dimension of my fitness plan into my daily routine. As I've stated in the past, brisk walking outdoors is one of the best things you can do for your body and state of mind. It stimulates the senses and creates an inner energy.

Usually I walk at a very fast pace for about 25 minutes or what turns out to be about 32 blocks. This little ritual helps me in many ways. For one, it gives my lungs a chance to breathe clean air, since most of my journey is done through Central Park. No matter who you are, or where you live, walking out in nature is better than walking on a treadmill, breathing in the stale recycled air of a crowded building. This walk I take also helps my cardiovascular system by elevating my heart rate, since I take long and deliberate (but quick) strides. As I pace through the park, I also meditate on the beauty of my surroundings—tall, lush trees, beautiful fields and meadows, meticulously kept gardens, the majestic Manhattan skyline, and the many bridges, stone walls, buildings and fountains that architects have constructed over the city's long, storied history. In the park, I truly have a chance to connect to nature, as well as to my physical and spiritual self.

Lastly, as I approach the gym, I begin to visualize how the workout will go— on which muscles I will be concentrating. In short, walking is a great ritual, multidimensional in its benefits, as you can see. I advise participating in a good, rigorous walk in nature 2–3 times a week.

During this ritual I also get to see other people enjoying themselves— rollerblading, running, biking, skateboarding...there is energy all around. The other morning, I slowed for a moment to observe a group of schoolchildren playing just behind one of the art museums. It was obviously a class outing and the kids were nearly bursting with energy. I mean, every single child was at full-throttle, nonstop. Not a single still or quiet body in the lot. Running, jumping, arms flailing in the air, screaming – aimless, chasing bodies in chaotic patterns. An absolute frenzy of poetic motion.

As I continued along, I started asking myself a few simple questions about what I had observed, and what the physical and possible metaphysical components behind the answers might be. The first, most obvious question was: Where does all that energy come from in young children? Certainly all those youngsters could not have been on special "energy" diets, like so many adults try. I mean, let's be serious, most kids I know eat very poorly– candy, soda, pizza, hot dogs and ice cream in large quantities, every day. These choices would add up to the antithesis of an energetic day for an adult.

Secondly, why weren't at least a few of these kids off in a corner somewhere being still? Certainly, amongst 50–60 adults, you would find at least a handful acting far less energized.

To answer the first question, we have to refer to the group of aging mechanisms and their counterparts, the biological markers of aging that I have written about so often. What is the number one known mechanism behind cellular level aging? Insulin resistance. Remember that insulin resistance is the hardening of the cell membrane. Insulin, primarily a storage hormone, loses its ability to store nutrients in the cell as the cell becomes more and more rigid, and less penetrable. This occurs over time, primarily because of an abundance of insulin itself, released from the pancreas in order to store and regulate glucose, often from refined foods and empty calories from "man-made" products. (Saturated fat is also a key contributor to insulin resistance).

Unfortunately, if we overeat or eat too many high-glycemic carbohydrates, a larger amount of insulin is secreted, both to store extra calories and balance blood glucose. As we do this continually, our blood sugar levels become disrupted because excessive amounts of food (and especially, refined food) push insulin levels up, while constantly driving blood sugar down. Energy is slowly lost, especially when cortisol is produced in order to hammer blood glucose down when insulin can no longer do so.

In an almost unconscious (yet feeble) attempt to restore blood glucose, most people reach for higher-glycemic carbohydrates, which in turn induce the pancreas to make more insulin, driving blood sugar levels down even more. This becomes a vicious cycle—energy is never fully restored. This is why so many people in our country become hypoglycemic and/or diabetic long before other aging markers occur. By this stage of the game, cultivating energy is a confusing, if not lost, function of one's body.

If you are an average American, eating lots of food (and lots of carbohydrates) over the course of 40 years or so, it will begin a cascading effect with other hormonal systems; feedback loops in the hypothalamus are negatively influenced by high glucose and/or high insulin levels. The hypothalamus is responsible for messages sent to the pituitary gland (amongst others), which controls the regulation of growth hormone and messages sent to the testes to secrete testosterone. The more these feedback loops are negatively affected by insulin and/or higher levels of glucose, the faster you will lose hormonal communication. The less hormonal communication you have, the faster you lose precious energy and speed up aging.

Not only will growth hormone, testosterone and other important hormones no longer be made in abundance as they were at the youthful stage, but what little is produced will not have the ability to penetrate cells (which have become hormonal and insulin resistant). Cyclic AMP, the important "second messenger" with the special "code" to unlock cell walls, will not be able to perform its task as well because of high levels of insulin and/or blood glucose. Get the picture? In part, we lose energy because of how we have chosen to eat. As Jerry Seinfeld once said in his stand-up routine, "I had one thought when I was young: 'Get candy!' " However, this has negative consequences down the road, as you can see.

As I continued my walk, I realized that if these (and all) children were taught about the real facts of nutrition and its influences on the body, they would be able to keep this type of energy a lot longer—assuming they chose the proper foods and quantities. Unfortunately, most of us do not learn about the intricacies and scientific aspects of nutrition until we start losing energy and questioning our own habits. Much of the damage has already been done by then. Of those 60 or so 10-year-olds I saw that day, many will have severe health problems by the time they reach my age (early 40s), and a good percentage of those health problems will be influenced by how those children eat over the course of their lives. A good deal of that precious energy will be taken away by poor eating habits. This is an absolute abomination, because scientists and nutritionists understand these aging mechanisms very well; yet, most of these kids (and their parents) will be influenced more by clever marketing techniques than they will by obscure scientific facts.

There was another lesson learned from this walk: energy, although primarily cultivated within (with proper nutrition and, to a lesser degree, one's state of mind), can be contagious. The fact that all these children were so engaged leads me to believe that outdoor recreation with others is not only fun—it is critical. Vitality is both physiologically and psychologically individual and communal. This is why I am such a big advocate of team sports, just as I am an advocate of working out with weights. Some of each is ideal.

The lesson here is simple: If you want to have youthful energy, eat a balanced diet with low-glycemic carbohydrates, walk in nature, train with weights, and find yourself a group of people (or a team) with whom to run around and have innocent fun. Your glory days will come marching back.

One other thing: If you are a parent, or thinking of being a parent, read as much as you can about nutrition and exercise. These two dimensions will have the biggest influence on your child's energy levels over the course of his/her lifetime. Perhaps there will be a day when a 40-year-old will have the endless energy of a child, thanks to anti-aging technology.

– Excerpted from *Exercise For Men Only* (Paul Burke's Over-40 Fitness Column)

———

FINDING THE "TRUTH"

Now, let's get back to the "here and now." After reading that article, you may pause to reflect on how you grew up and how your parents also ate what they were taught to eat by their parents and how one can trace this all the way back to a certain point in history. From that point moving backward, however, there is only anthropology and archeology which informs us about what our greatest ancestors ate and why. That certain point is where I will begin the actual text of this book, and then I will go forward slowly into today's nutritional (sorry to say) nightmare and how it got to be that dark and horrifying monster that we are (almost) all consuming. All of what I have written over the course of this entire book are chapters based on the knowledge which I have gained over multiple years of competition, training others, receiving my undergraduate and graduate degrees, and studying on my own. I have learned by studying everything I could find about our evolution, by going to the New York City Natural History Museum, by taking critical thinking courses on religion and theology, by human trial and error, and through pure logic deduced from the tower of books which I have studied about evolution, aboriginal culture nutrition, the advent of plant and animal domestication, and food refinement and processing.

In all of my books and published articles, I always say that I am a logician first before a health major, exercise physiologist, professor, or professional trainer. The reason behind this is that despite Emanuel Kant's phenomenal book, *The Critique of Pure Reason*, logic is not reason. Logic can only be agreed upon and tested with facts and the "*knowing of truths*."

The paradox of "real" logic is that on the one hand you may actually progress into ascertaining certain data which can predict certain outcomes; on the other hand, you know that all logic is most solid when based in experiential learning and observation. I had a brilliant philosophy professor tell me once that science is flawed, as are the sciences of many didactically taught vocations (such as MDs, PhDs, psychologists, and so on). He believed that no one could be truly "objective" and that logic and truth are not mutually exclusive, nor are they mutually bound, until you become more and more *subjective*. In other words, until you have tried everything yourself, reflected upon it deeply, and really embodied it, you cannot base any logical argument for or against something. Thus, all of those books and titles which I have read, reflected upon, and absorbed may have been written by those who were taught via didactic learning. However, a true logician learns through experience, reflection, and subjective observation, and even the subjective *imagination* (or meditation) of putting one into the past - not only through what is written or what is seen "objectively" by others, but also by way of knowing intrinsically. I have learned that what is written is a good place to start the inquiry of a specific area of interest, but it is not a place to end learning, nor are good books and great professors the means to an end. A book of any knowledge is only as good as the experiences which the author has been willing to try before writing. These subjective experiences are the deepness which is missing in our world today. When someone does this deep subjective thinking and reflection, they are said to be "*thinking out of the box*," and I would say that only in the sense that the box represents a certain set of pretenses made by man, to either make money or to take control (of society).

Ironically, the very thing which we can totally control and should experience in our lives, most choose not to control or not to exercise caution about what they put into their mind and body. If food did not make a difference in the outcome of one's life, health, liberty, and the pursuit of happiness, then there wouldn't be so many diet books and so many failed dieters. If you eat as I have learned to eat, any number of miracles will begin to take place. I give you my word on this - my deepest and most empathetic word.

As I mentioned, in order to understand anything in life, one actually must become more and more "subjective" as opposed to what many scientists term "objective," because there simply is no such thing as total "objective observation." All observation is skewed with that which each lens has been glossed over through experiences. Since this has been proven by everyone from Kant to Albert Einstein, I have gone through life reading, studying, and "doing." This "doing of things" not only includes experimentations which I have done on myself, but also on others. Thus, I "know"— the greater part of the word "know-ledge" ("the knowing of")—what appears to be the truth. I cannot—with the ethical and moral standards which I have been determined to stick to all of my adult life—write or endorse anything which I do not believe in myself. In order to believe in something, I must firstly, therefore, do it myself before I instruct others to do so. This is where I find it difficult to understand the logic in the so-called "health care system." The average doctor lives to be fifty-eight years old in the United States. The doctors to whom I refer are often the only people who instruct many of us about our health—what "we" (the collective public consciousness) should be eating and how we should be monitoring our lifestyle, heart health, glucose levels, and so forth. I know only a handful of doctors who understand and act upon the proper lifestyle which is so important. The others simply do not know, nor do they seemingly care to know, what history has taught humans for eons of time. The food which our pre-agrarian ancestors ate was the food which made us become *Homo sapiens*, and yet we choose to ignore what they ate and why they ate it. Instead, we eat a diet filled with refined foods, and we have a hugely profitable, infrequently mentioned agricultural industry which procures more of what we should *not* eat. If you read on, I will inform you about the answers to the questions of the *when,* the *what,* the *why,* and the *why not* of human nutrition.

A logician tries very hard to understand facts and the historical value about which those facts inform him/her in order to concretize what was once a human "intuition." Yet so many people's eyes (and thus conscious understanding) have been glossed over by everything from "inventions of food" to clever marketing and political lobbying. You may not realize that what you are (more than likely) eating has little to do with physiological correctness and healthiness for you and your children. Rather, it is the result of how well lobbyists and didactically taught doctors and (some) nutritionists have used their political power to influence the masses to keep items such as wheat-based (and other grain-based) foods on the market, complete with sports stars and Olympians on the front of the boxes of just a minor portion of the wheat-based and grain-based foods which we consume. I can't think of a more destructive thing to do than to eat wheat products (refined, as they all are) day after day for a lifetime.

This idea of politics is not to say that all of these people are involved in some type of grand conspiracy; rather, they are teaching what they have been taught. The problem lies herein—the students, as with the teachers, cannot see the trees beyond the forest, and cannot make a truthful decision because they have been led by blind faith in a system that doesn't think in terms of health, but rather in terms of dollars and cents and what is most cost-effective. They have not studied the body's historical nutritional dilemmas and paradoxes, nor have most of them actually practiced what evolution teaches.

Having said that, I honestly believe that most people have what they believe is the "truth" on their side and, therefore, should not be judged; however, in order to find the "one and only" truly human nutritional understanding, all one has to do is to spend a lifetime (as I have) exploring everything from the origin of thought to the consciousness of the human mind and its ability to separate us from the rest of the wild animal world and even distinguish us from other mammals. (Or you can merely read this book, and you will have all of the knowledge and tools with which to guide you as to how to eat and why.)

I have always tried to right the wrongs and protect the rights of truth. Truth is not what is on a television commercial or written on the side of a cereal box. Instead, truth lies within our genes, within our cells, within our DNA, within our deepest consciousness, within our evolution. Truth, I surmise, is when one reaches the highest level of consciousness which one can about any one subject - that level of consciousness which all other living things on this wonderful earth "know" without thought and without anything other than intuitively following action and reaction to the sun, water, earth, and fire. Their action and reaction to this world and the simplistic evidence (put forth in this book) is usually difficult to find amongst the myriad of consumer marketing ploys and the buzzwords of the nutritional supplements and dietary world. We find ourselves making the simple complex, while reducing the complexity into fractions and decimal points of mechanistic compartmentalization. When it comes to nutrition, however, even the smartest of humans seems to fall prey to "diets." As this book infers, there can be only one "human diet," and that really isn't a "diet" at all—rather, it is a simple "miracle" of truth in the past, present, and for the future. This is a group of nuggets of wisdom amongst chocolate cake and "whole wheat bread" (as if there could ever be such a thing as whole-wheat bread—it's been refined into dust before adding leavening ingredients and other chemicals).

The nutritional pillars of our history, ancestry, and our evolution are all included in this book. The pillars which I discuss are those which have given us the ability to keep cells fresh and young, and to keep the body evolving and living longer for each advancing millennium. However, a certain group of what may be called "brilliant" inventions brought these pillars all the way down to the ground, now and perhaps forever, unless you take the knowledge in this book and use it to guide you and your loved ones forever more.

This diet is all based on the *how, what,* and *why* we eat as we do, and *how, what,* and *why* we should eat as I have written in this book. It is not a secret or some celebrity's idea of a "diet;" rather, it is the only healthy, non-addictive, *human* way to eat! As you read this book, you will see the *when,* the *what,* the *how,* and the *why* of this diet which is as old as the last true hunter-gatherer aboriginals of the entire globe. As Socrates, the first great "civil" teacher, once said, "*A life not reflected upon is a life not worth living.*" What I believe this says to us in this sense is that we "know" what is good for our bodies and what is not; however, many choose to fool themselves into thinking contrarily, all for the sake of taste instead of nutritional sense and needs.

It is my hope that mothers, fathers, sons, and daughters will read this, talk about it, and reflect upon the truths and the falsehoods/fakes - the "faux-foods," a term I have coined and about which I have often written. Only then can you make a truly informed decision on the way to a healthy way of eating. There is no gimmickry at work here—just the facts, Jack, just the facts.

I welcome you all into my world of nutritional truth. There is no disputing the facts of our past, our organic evolution, the biological markers of aging, nor the miracles which I have seen once one takes up a diet such as that written about in this book. There is no disputing our disconnection from the very fundamental ideals that once were the nutritional staple of every human on the face of this earth— which has sadly become a place permeated by commercialism and foods which are as addictive as cocaine. Yes, I wrote what you read. Refined foods (flours, sugars, and other refined, manipulated, and processed foods) are as addictive as cocaine. This is where we have strayed way off course; however, it is not the key disruption – rather, it is the distance between what was once "wild" and what became "domesticated" which changed human evolution forever.

Once you understand certain concepts here, you too will experience the loss of addiction and gain wisdom—wisdom which was once as automatic to every human as is blinking. I suggest that you read this book closely so that if you do blink, you won't miss a word or misinterpret the major process which our great ancestors all went through in order for us to have the world we have today, yet without a lot of what any person who has studied this would call a travesty at best and a marketing supreme killing machine. Unfortunately, there have been so many problems created by our superior "intelligence," marketing, and consumerism, that there are few humans who can live far enough away from commercialism to understand what it has done to humans' brains and their food consumption. Fortunately, I have been able to see the forest and the trees, to live outside the boundaries of cultural commercialism and politics, and to understand what this one miracle is, this one "human" diet.

You too must go back into the early stages of human evolution with me. You will, all of a sudden, realize that all the time the truth of nutrition was staring you right in the face while your consumer-driven blinders prevented you from seeing that truth. I hope that this book helps as many people as possible to remove the blinders and "see" the truth of nutrition for the first time. It is up to you whether you follow this "One Human Diet." It is always up to you.

———

CHAPTER I

A BRIEF HISTORY OF HUMAN FOOD CONSUMPTION

CARNIVORES, OMNIVORES, AND SPECIALISTS

No matter where you go for your anthropological (and/or archeological) knowledge, all of the anthropologists and paleo-nutritionologists whom I have read agree that we became the thinking, conscious, handy-humans at about the same time, worldwide, for the very same reasons, and it was *de novo*—"without influence." Anthropologists call this era "*The Great Leap Forward*." Part of the human evolution during "*The Great Leap*" some 40,000 years ago was that communications, creativity, and innovative mobility began to take up (and make) more and more brain space; suddenly (in terms of evolution), our organs (such as the pancreas, liver, and kidneys, etc.) all stopped evolving. That means our organs froze in evolutionary time. Whatever was being eaten at that time, therefore, would become the way of the future—the only way one would and could survive. A brilliant yet paradoxically horrific set of nutritional changes would be humanly devised some 30,000 years into the future of these Paleolithic (and forward, Neo-Paleolithic) beings. Let's take a short history course in how humans ate in those early days of our ancestry as Paleolithic, then Neo-Paleolithic, and finally Neolithic humans so as to begin to roll the blinders back to see the truth of what gave us our endlessly utilitarian brain ability along with an ancient body—but one that any bodybuilder would be proud to bring to the stage in this new millennium. (Or, as my academic mentor would say, "*Peel away the onion layers that are so painfully hiding the center, the center of truth, and these layers do so much so that one cries all the way to that center, where we see truth for the first time and are set, as Dr. Martin Luther King so eloquently said, 'Free at last! Free at last! Thank God Almighty, we are free at last!'*") No, this is not a book about race, per se; although, all of my studies have brought me to believe that we are all the same, all from the same hominoids (proto-humans), all coming from the same place—Africa. What we would eat along our journey of walking this sphere which we have named "Earth" is what I am interested in, for this will set you free, too—free from dieting, free from roller-coaster eating, free from the addiction that all refined and/or grain-based foods cause. Let us look back—to the earliest days of our closest ancestors.

THE EVOLUTION OF HUMAN FOOD CONSUMPTION

Early humans in the years preceding plant and animal domestication (10,000 to 2,500 years ago, depending upon where you look) were all hunter-gatherers. There is no question about this. Anthropologists and archeologists all agree with this "truth." I have studied and meditated upon all the tremendous amount of work and detail that others before me have left behind for all of us to read and utilize, for no truer words have ever been uttered than those who merely say that "*the future lies in the details of the past.*" Thus, there is nothing in this book that is "made up" or "supernatural." It is all based on the endless amounts of information provided by passionate men and women who have spent lifetimes piecing together the long chain of human history—link by painstaking link. In this case, the history of human food consumption is where we want to begin our thoughts.

The more which you can absorb relative to our ancestors' evolution, the greater the chances are that you will grasp the concepts of nutrition, aging, and health which are revealed in this book. Everything that is "right" for our bodies can still be found if you know where to look. The key is to understand *why* we should eat this certain way which will be revealed as you read. People come up with clever ideas for diets, but no one ever seems to do enough homework to convince a majority of the people that food which was once a natural source of all the nutritional elements needed is really right in front of all of us. We have been conned into thinking that a special and unique "gimmick" is our magic bullet to achieve slim, trim, and ageless bodies; however, it is the exact opposite of what many diet books say.

The earliest ancestors of ours ate whatever, whenever they could. During our early evolution, three major but distinct groups of hominoids (proto-humans) were pushed out of the jungles of Africa because of a massive geological change of weather patterns, especially on that particular continent. These distinct groups of proto-humans took various routes of travel from their origins and thus took up various forms of eating, which accordingly depended upon what they found on their route out of Africa to various destinations. These destinations are what we know today as Western Europe, the Middle East, and the Far East (or *Asia*). One thing is for certain—without an ocean to divide the enormous land mass of what we know as *Eurasia*, these proto-humans spread over this entire area from Africa up into Europe and eastward to China within a relatively short period of time.

The group we are primarily interested in is the one which survived and would later become *Homo sapiens*, our ancestors. The other two major groups died off because they were what paleo-nutritionologists call "specialists." These specialists tried to survive on a diet of mostly leaves (a few other roots and/or fruits for some). By remaining frugivores (fruit eaters) and/or folivores (leaf eaters), they perished within a matter of years. To these frugivores and folivores, hunting was unheard of because they were either surrounded by vegetation, or they did not have the know-how to hunt. Because of this, they ate leaves and (some) fruit. Proto-humans who were folivores or frugivores, then, all died off eons ago. We had evolved past the ape stage, past the stage of dragging our knuckles on the ground—and amazingly, these proto-humans had become a new species. However, trying to find the proper food during this phase of evolution was very difficult.

Homo sapiens added meat to their diet and became carnivorous omnivores as they found their way around the world—on foot. They continued to grow both physically and mentally as they made weapons to hunt, and thus were able to kill and eat wild animals, often eating their catch raw. (Cooking food was done in some tribes; however, originally, everyone ate their food raw). They also gathered wild vegetables, *wild* grains, wild roots, wild nuts, wild berries, and often wild fruits and edible leaves. This all took great strength, effort, teamwork, raw speed, and power to hunt down the huge animals of the day and to find wild roots, berries, and nuts—all scattered around the forests and outer edges of barren open spaces in the new lands into which *Homo sapiens* walked. (I believe in the lure of the never-ending horizon—the sun that continually gave them light, life, and that wonderful feeling which we all get when we see the sunset, reflecting upon today and looking forward to tomorrow). I believe that the shape of the earth (a sphere) was alluring to those who chose to chase that magnificent and endless horizon which never seemed to be accessible, yet it kept these people moving around the globe. Our main question here is what was being eaten during these days of spanning the sphere of the earth?

The human powerhouses who walked this entire earth for the first time were called the (Upper and Middle) Paleolithians, Neo-Paleolithians, and eventually "Neolithians." They were seasonally nomadic and constantly on the move, doing daily tasks and tracking the herds of animals that were their food, their deity, and their clothing. They often moved for hundreds of miles on foot in horrendous conditions. Finding food was a daily ritual which took on religious[1] proportions. Even the "chief" of any tribe had to find his *own* food.

Besides the mythologies which were driven by the intrinsic feelings of being part of nature and giving reverence to the main hunted mammal, it also took great intelligence to coordinate "the hunt." To track, locate, and kill the giant animals - which would be eaten and used for almost every item in their lives - was a task made for big, fast, powerful men. This intelligence and innate knowledge of how humans made and used actual weapons for hunting is unique in all of mammalian evolution. The key here is that our ancestors survived because of this intuitive intelligence and because they hunted and ate wild game, and gathered and ate wild vegetables, wild grains, wild roots, wild nuts, and wild berries. *Wild, wild,* and *wild*; and *whole, whole, whole*[2]. The human body evolved while eating whole, wild, raw food. Do not eat raw

---

1   The word "religion" comes from the Latin word "*religio*," which means to "link back to." All early indigenous cultures believed that their main food source was their deity. For more on this, see "Notes."

2   Foods were eaten whole. Our pancreas and other organs evolved to eat wild and whole foods.

wild meat now, or you will keel over and drop dead of something. However, do learn that everything is meant to be eaten "whole, raw (if possible), and wild." That is how we were eating at the time when our organs *stopped* evolving.[3] What are the foods of today which best mimic those of our super-athletic, super-strong ancestors? Read on, my friends—it will come to you in time, just as it did for them.

The most important two parts of our early ancestry to remember are how we evolved and what we ate during that time and thereafter (until a very specific time in our ancient history, which, as I have stated, is when our organs stopped evolving). That time is roughly 40,000 years ago when we had completely organically evolved. All of our mastication acids, all of our hormonal organs, the hypothalamus, pituitary, *pancreas*, kidneys, spleen—all of our organs stopped organically evolving about 40,000 years ago. This means that by 38,000 BC, our organs stopped evolving because we had stabilized on this carnivorous and omnivorous diet of wild meat, whole wild plants, whole wild roots, whole wild vegetables, whole wild fruits, wild nuts, and wild fish in certain areas. This is extremely important to remember—everything eaten by our early ancestors was wild and was usually eaten whole.

---

3   Everyone who has become known as an authority on anthropological (and to some extent archeological) studies believes that organs stopped evolving in the human body 40,000 years ago. This is a key note to understand. Our brains did not stop evolving, nor our musculoskeletal systems—just our organs. The pancreas is the most important organ to remember in this brief history of our ancestral nutrition.

CHAPTER II

THE CHANGING OF THE GUARD IN HUMAN EVOLUTION

Our ancestors participated in the aforementioned lifestyle until somewhere between 10,000 and 2,500 years ago, depending on the location of the tribe. At this period in history, the world changed for humans in every conceivable way. Slowly but surely, the brain became so "intelligent" because our earliest ancestors had used their hands to crush and crack open the skulls of carcasses left behind by wild carnivores and ate the brains of all types of animals. In those brains were loads of DHA and DEA—two important fatty acids which are needed for outer cortex construction. In other words, we became "physiologically intelligent" in part because our earliest ancestors survived by eating the "leftovers" of a kill by another wild animal. Actual intelligence is postulated to have come from the earliest of these hunters beginning to contemplate their ability and great use of their hands.[4] These two developments, one physiological and one metaphysical, were the two main reasons for brain growth, human intelligence, self-awareness, and consciousness.

Our earliest ancestors used their thumbs and fingers, their amazing hands (which they passed along to us with amazing dexterity), to smash the skulls of carcasses and eat the brains of the mammal left behind by huge carnivores which could not eat anything inside the skull—for they did not have the hands and dexterity to do so. This was the beginning of our physiological "brain" as we know it today. It took both this physiological construct together with *contemplation* about the hand's ability which began the chain of events which led us to the ability to "think." Because of the development of our brains and our hands, no other mammal on earth can do the necessary and progressive steps which it took to evolve as we did. Our only endlessly evolving organ is our brain.

---

4   E. O. Wilson, a professor and highly-respected author at Harvard University, believes that had our hand not evolved as one with great dexterity, we never would have evolved beyond the state of being hominoids (proto or pre-human). See "Notes" for more.

During the post Neo-Paleolithic and the turn of the Neolithic era, the beginning of a process that would later be known as animal and plant domestication began. Evolution and human dietary habits took on a new course, as you shall see.

The six most commonly agreed upon areas in the world where this type of living had its origins are the Fertile Crescent (8,500 BC), China (7,500 BC), Central and Southern Mexico (3,000 BC), Central America and the Andes of South America (3,000 BC), possibly the Amazon Basin (3,000 BC), and the eastern region of the United States (2,500 BC).[5]

It is believed that each of these areas above (with the exception of Europe and North America) began food domestication and production *de novo* (without influence from each other), using the indigenous plants and animals which were easiest to replicate and/or tame, corral, plant, and domesticate ("domesticated" means raised near the "home"). These were not simple matters; rather, it required tremendous creative intelligence which would rival any rocket scientist or neurosurgeon of today. In fact, the long and arduous tasks of figuring out which wild plants and wild grains could be replanted and replicated in fields of grain, which animals could be bred together, or how to make a wild animal become domesticated, was not easy for our ancestors. We have to remember the setting of the time. Wild game began to become increasingly hard to find for each and every tribe on earth. This is mostly because they hunted them all to near extinction over many thousands of years. In addition, finding or hunting for food before food domestication, *was* a person's vocation and religion, a "linking back" to ancestral roots. Whether you were a chief or a person without any bloodline to power, everyone was either a hunter or a gatherer until plant and animal domestication, which not only changed nutrition, but also changed the way in which our ancestors and future people would live.

With wild animals becoming harder to find in many areas, especially in those areas which were the first to domesticate food—that is, the Fertile Crescent (the area which we call Iraq today) and parts of Asia—the people of these areas were quick to domesticate certain animals and certain (plant) crops for convenience in order that they would have time to do other things in life besides hunting and gathering food each day. This may seem like a logical step to take, and it was; however, it is the very process of how wild plants and wild animals were domesticated which would turn evolution upside down forever.

As time passed and they made some very interesting observations about nature, men (and probably women in concert) began to realize that plant and animal domestication was possible. It would be the weakest of plants, however, which would begin to change the once magnificent specimens of the Paleolithic, Neo-Paleolithic, and Neolithic eras—through a slow declination in musculoskeletal structure—into the fat and short Europeans of the era of King Henry VIII. Then, in the late nineteenth and mid-twentieth centuries, some height and musculature was gained back—which

---

5   Taken from Jared Diamond's phenomenal Pulitzer Prize winning non-fiction book, *Guns, Germs, and Steel.* See "Notes" for more.

we have reason to believe was because of the generous amount of calories nearly every person was able to either buy or raise on their farms. That was about nine inches of height lost on each human in six to eight millennia—from the time directly before plant and animal domestication to the early to mid-eighteenth century. The male body especially shrunk both in height and muscle mass. Oddly, those indigenous (or what we now call aboriginal) cultures on each continent still retained some height and more lean muscle because they stayed with both hunting and gathering with only some domestication. (A small bell should be waking you up now—something should be ticking inside your brain, telling you at least part of your missing link to the "right food" and which foods cause problems).

THE FUNDAMENTALS OF ANCIENT PLANT DOMESTICATION

Of all the potential edible foliage in the world, only 1 percent is fit for human consumption. It took many thousands of years to know which plants could be domesticated for human consumption and even more time for humans to become observant enough of nature to make the drastic move from hunter-gatherers to domesticated plant and animal farmers. Some groups domesticated earlier than others, probably due to the respective availability of food and their placement on the globe. For instance, those who were equatorial cultures never needed to domesticate plants because there was such a natural abundance of vegetation.[6] Those, however, who lived along what we have called the Fertile Crescent started agrarianism much sooner because of the geographical climate and the number of people who had evolved in that area of the world.

Once the natural supply of wild game, plants, and fruits began to diminish within an area, an effort had to be made to find new ways of procuring food. Prior to this, a scarcity of food merely meant it was time to move the tribe on to better hunting grounds and new forests where fruits, roots, and berries would be more plentiful, as would wild game. At some point, depending on necessity, larger tribes realized that they could raise one or two crops of edible plants, store them, and then eat

6   As stated, the species that survived and thrived were the carnivorous omnivores, and although those living around the equator did rely on vegetation, they too loved to hunt small animals and eat them just as some indigenous cultures still do. This is the evolutionary evidence that the human body was not designed to be vegetarian as some radical-thinking people would have you believe. Has our game supply changed? Yes, it has, and that is why we must try to limit grain-raised red meat and chicken. What we should look for are "pastured" animals and wild fish and free-range chickens which are free of hormones and antibiotics. You can safely say now, without question, that to become a vegetarian is by choice, not by design. As the famous mythologist and archeologist Joseph Campbell used to say, "Those who are vegetarians are merely running from the fact that life eats life and has done so since the dawn of our existence." See "Notes" for more on Campbell.

when necessary; this was much more efficient than wandering through the woods looking for wild vegetation and animals to kill each day. Observing events around them—such as the fact that melons grew from seeds in piles of hyena feces (in parts of Africa, hyenas all go to the same area to defecate)—may have helped early "farmers" (still hunter-gatherers) realize that not only could they grow fruit from the seeds found in the fruit, but also that animal feces may help fertilize the crop's growth. Seeds, it turns out, have a protective coating around them, and this was a uniquely evolved procreative device which allows the seeds to be carried in the stomach and intestines of any mammal or reptile. This can move the seeds into a new area for rooting—once the seed passes through that mammal via defecation. Then procreation-transport began in new areas for any particular vegetation with seeds. It may be merely by coincidence, then, that hyenas of Africa ate melons and all defecated in one single pile, and then humans observed wild melons growing in the spring and summer from this pile. A new awareness was realized, nonetheless, that seeds were meant to be planted to make more new fruit. Fruits then made seeds which had also morphed, in their evolution, in such a way so that no matter who or what ate them, there would be a new home for procreation. This is how fruits (and other seed-bearing vegetation) with seeds ensured species survivability. This is most important to note, for it will bring us closer to understanding other man-made "manipulations" of natural selection within evolution.

Early plant domestication would change the evolution of plants through the clever examinations of very observant people who would one day be called "farmers." For example, wild almonds were once all deadly poisonous. The intensely bitter taste from an almond comes from amygdalin, which breaks down into the lethal gas cyanide. In the natural almond tree, one or two trees out of thousands contain a genetic mutation which prevents them from producing amygdalin, and the almonds from these trees are "sweet" edible almonds. However, birds and animals could and did eat these almonds, putting the mutated trees at a disadvantage in evolutionary terms. These trees would never make it to procreation, for their mutation had to be wiped out, and nature had a method for this. Other species would eat these mutant seeds, and the poisonous almonds would remain intact as a total species. That tiny mutant population would be destroyed by other species, ensuring the procreation of only poisonous trees to keep the species of almond trees alive and well.

Since the seeds from these trees were being eaten, none of the trees with the mutation were being reproduced. Thus the species remained intact as it had evolved—with poisonous fruit.

Early humans observed birds and other animals eating these sweet almonds from a tiny group out of hundreds of thousands of poisonous almond trees. With their intelligence, powers of conjecture, and newfound agrarian skills, humans realized that they could plant and grow these mutated almond seeds which would produce sweet nuts instead of poisonous ones. This was evolution disruption number one.

Thus the process of natural selection, which would normally have exterminated a mutation of this type, had been interrupted by humans' ability to selectively grow these mutated trees from seeds they had gathered, thereby creating an entire crop of mutant plants. Today, almost all almond trees are sweet and are thus a batch of mutated trees.

Another clear example of humans altering the course of plant evolution can be understood by mapping the progression of the little green pea. In the wild, when the peas are ripe, the pod explodes, and peas are dispersed all around the outlying area to grow new plants. However, in as many as 0.2–5.0 percent of these plants, the pods *do not* explode. Normally, the peas from these defective plants would die entombed in their pods, withering away in the late summer sun. However, early on in our history, humans took the seeds from these mutant pea plants and planted them in order that the harvest of the peas would be easier and more efficient than scrambling in the dirt for each single pea from the exploding pod. Those pods which were *not* mutated were the ones which exploded. In these wild pea plants, the exploded seeds were the ones which procreated—just as evolution intended. Once again, human intervention saved a mutant plant from extinction and changed the course of evolution by planting mutant seeds which would make rows of peas created from one or two mutant plants (in the dawn of human plant domestication).

Wheat and barley, two of the most widely used crops in the world today, in their wild state drop their seeds when their stalks "shudder," and the wind helps scatter the strongest of the seeds to ensure procreation remains intact. This shuddering ability is an evolutionary development to aid in the spreading of the seeds from these wild grains. There are mutated plants on which the stalk *does not* shudder, and thus the seeds stay on the plant. In the wild, this mutation would soon disappear because these seeds would not have the advantage of the seeds which get spread on the ground—blown by the wind into a virgin area to root. However, humans once again observed this and saw the benefit of keeping the seeds from the stalks which did not shudder, so they saved them for planting and harvesting and thus decided to plant and grow seeds from these mutated plants. Over thousands of years of this process, we now have wheat and barley fields entirely made up of once-mutant seeds from once-mutant plants. There is only 10–20 percent of the world's population which does not have some type of negative reaction to wheat, barely, and/or all other domestic grains. It is not merely that they were made from mutated plants, however. The organs in the body had long ago (30,000–40,000 years ago to be exact) stopped evolving, and the large amounts of these once wild plants (now grown in large domesticated fields of grain) which we began to consume, was a huge shock to the already steady pancreatic response to wild grains, wild fruits, and berries. This would then begin a long line of progressively intolerable foods made from these ever-growing crops of mutated wheat seeds and other grain seeds. Soon, some 9,750 years into the future, there would be the invention of the gristmill, food processing, and refined wheat and other grains taken down to mere powder which would be called "flour." This is where it all began to go terribly wrong for the human body. Few people know that a mere one in ten people can even tolerate any type of grain and that these few people have what is known as a "blunted" insulin response to processed grains such as pasta, whole wheat bread, bagels, crackers, cookies, and any other type of food made from grain products. In other words: STOP EATING ANYTHING MADE FROM GRAINS. The body simply did not evolve while eating these domesticated grains and super-sugars known as granular flours. Therefore, they cause inflammation at the least, and food allergies, chronic illness, diabetes, and yes, you guessed it, cell death at the worst. If you eat enough grain-based foods, your cells will age three times as fast as if you had eaten whole fruits, whole vegetables, nuts, and lean, "pastured," non-steroidal/non-growth-hormone *wild* chicken, wild turkey, and wild oily fish.

So, between 2,000 and 10,000 years ago, humans began eating a diet consisting of mutated plants and domesticated animals (about which I will give details shortly). Since the body had evolved eating *wild* plants and *wild* animals, the pancreatic response alone was much more aggressive with any type of grains which were domesticated; later in history, refined foods - as I mentioned – are enough to overwhelm cells to death ("resistance" to the storage hormone insulin). Until man had made many other refinements to these mutated plants which eventually took on such names as "amber waves of grain," these domesticated grains were merely shrinking the musculoskeletal system; however, now that these grains have been refined, they are causing 80–90 percent of the American population to have severe health issues. No such problem ever existed on earth until we humans manipulated nature and developed an entire industry, an actual lifeline for the world to survive on, cheaply raised and harvested grains. I can say with total confidence that anything made with grains today is detrimental to your health.

Within a very short period of time, man changed evolution by domesticating the very plants intended to be plucked out by evolution, the trees and plants that normally would have been wiped out by nature because they were defective. Clearly, this was a zenith of human creativity, and yet it was about to give our intelligence, which enabled this marvel of crop-raising, its greatest paradoxical problematic move forward. Man had changed evolution and all the world's cultures forever. Not only had man changed the evolution of these once wild plants, but he would inevitably become craftier and would design such technological marvels as the gristmill and other factories of refinement, as I have already mentioned. It would be these two hugely intelligent factors which would one day create an epidemic of type II diabetes and a plethora of other chronic illnesses—the largest of which is wheat and grain intolerance, food allergies and *sensitivities*—which often begin an autoimmune response if enough of these grains are given to certain humans.

The ultimate human paradox had been created. Out of need, man had engineered perhaps his greatest marvel—the domesticated plant and the ability to now have time for other activities, instead of searching for food every day. In the beginning, this was probably a fairly smart concept; it would change the world in every conceivable way over the next five to ten millennia. We would go from a man of 6'1" and 220 pounds of muscle, on average, to a man in seventeenth-century England who was a towering 5'6" tall, with a potbelly worthy of naming fat, iron stoves after. However, plant and animal domestication had more consequences. The lean body mass of a pre-agrarian hunter-gatherer would have been very high—as much as 95 percent of his body would have been heavily muscled, and skeletally and organically pure and free of saturated fat. Where might we have found the lean body mass index of the strongest man around in Europe in the 1600s? He would have had a paltry 60 percent lean muscle mass and a whopping 40 percent fat—saturated fat. Ah, but the truly deleterious, vicious wonders of plant and animal domestication were still four centuries away. Although the scourge of the "Black Plague" (caused by living too close to newly domesticated animals) would be the most overt problem which plant and animal domestication would inflict, the worst was yet to come. I shall save you from total despair until the other paradoxes have all been neatly aligned, in order that you too can understand how a once brilliant idea turned the entire world upside down.

THE FUNDAMENTALS OF ANIMAL DOMESTICATION

"There were only fourteen wild herbivores in the entire world that made it onto the domesticated list. Of those ancient fourteen, the "minor nine" are the Arabian, the Bactrian camel, the llama, the donkey, the reindeer, the water buffalo, the yak, the banteng, and the gaur. The remaining "major five" are the cow, sheep, goat, pig, and horse."[7] The cow as we know it today was domesticated by combining animals and altering breeding similar to the variations of dogs—all coming from one lone wolf pack. The American Indians (and other indigenous tribes all over the world) were some of the first tribal people who utilized the wolf for guarding the horses, and eventually they were the very people who domesticated them, with the wolves often guarding their masters from the United States Cavalry. (I will talk more about this concept later on in the book). Those animals which were domesticated for food are the ones which we want to watch right now, for they too would have a serious, profound, and lasting effect on the human species. (I will allow you to decide if that effect was worth it in terms of how it affected us as a species).

---

7   Taken verbatim from Jared Diamond's Pulitzer Prize winning book, *Guns, Germs, and Steel.*

Domesticated animals differ in many ways from their wild ancestors for two reasons:

1. Human selection and breeding to get the "best" results have changed the form and shape of these animals to suit humans' tastes, not nature's reality or her proclivity.
2. The vast automatic evolutionary response of animals to the artificial environment has altered the forces of natural selection to allow those animals who are better suited to such an environment to survive.

Domesticated animals have changed physiologically and organically from their original design as wild animals (or the wild animals which were mated into domestication). From their brains and muscle, to their organs, there is no question that these vital internal functionalities have slowly atrophied, just as ours have been disrupted over the millennia. You will soon be easily swayed to see how and why this happened.

With these changes has come a weakening of the domesticated animals which we (those of us who are carnivorous omnivores) now eat as everyday food. This adds to something which I go into later in the book regarding the actual (metaphysical) energy acquired from eating a cow which barely moves during its entire life and eats a mixture of grains and often drugs (such as cheap antibiotics, growth hormones, and other horrendous things). Compare this to eating a *wild* deer or elk, an animal which never stops moving every day of its life and eats nothing but *wild* food. Think about a herd of cows today—they are often chained in a metal stall-type fixture and are fed a daily mixture of grains, hay, and other additives such as antibiotics (for fattening), growth hormone, anabolic steroids for quickened mass production, and water which may or may not be fit for consumption. (Yes, even a cow can get sick from water toxicity due to pollutants or, even worse, mercury and other heavy metals—very toxic and often deadly to the human nervous system). The problem is that these cows cannot talk and tell us what it feels like to live a life such as this. They can't wave their hooves at the owner and say, "*This water tastes as if it is tainted with chemicals.*" I think you get the picture.

Most domesticated animals raised for regular grocery stores (and almost every different kind of food store, with a few exceptions) are raised chained to a stall, crammed in a coop, or worse. What we really have here is more of an auto-animal that is synthetically made, synthetically grown, and synthetically packaged. Not only are these animals fatter in content, but they are only one step removed from being something not of this earth. I am not one to be offensive to any person who raises or eats these animals, in the same way that many people are about certain furs and skins of other types of animals; rather, I am much more interested in, and intent upon, trying to educate the masses about what it is which they are consuming. Our pre-agrarian, massively muscular, athletic Paleolithic ancestor would not do well eating the species which we call a cow today. Guess what? Neither are we! Not only is what the cow eats getting into our body, but the energy (the utilization of the musculature of the cow or lack thereof) is also getting into our body via absorption through cellular uptake. There is no getting around the fact that we cannot go back to Paleolithic times and run around after wild deer each and every day; however, we can demand that our food supply be raised as wild, albeit *pastured,* domesticated animals. What does it take? It takes an extra three acres to raise cows the way that they were "designed" to be raised. Whoever thought of making an animal like a cow anyway? You must remember there is no such thing as a "wild" cow.

Now, just think about this for a moment. This cow is fed grains, which I have already concluded is not good for human consumption (based on not only grains' mutant ancestral path, but the fact that grains are a poor choice to make an animal healthy). We made the cows' organs shrink within five or six generations; that is like a blink of an eye in evolutionary terms. Yet despite the cow's horrific life, despite the enormous amount of saturated fat (which contributes to insulin resistance and arterial sclerosis), and despite the crippling diseases that cows would give to humans (thousands of years ago and ironically again today with the so called "mad cow disease"), we continue to turn these animals into nothing more than sitting sacks of saturated fat and marbleized protein. If you can get your beef organically raised, free-range and/or pastured, and without hormones and antibiotics, then you are a bit ahead of the game.

To come back to the metaphysical side of things, for I can hear my scientist friends now, energy is a big part of food consumption. However, few nutritionists give it any thought beyond the physical thermodynamics of caloric intake in the form of protein, carbohydrates, and fat which make up the macronutrients in dissection of what we eat when chewing on this wonderful, if nothing else, sad sack of organs, fat, and drugs. My belief about energy is that the more "wild" the energy inside the animal's parasympathetic and autonomic nervous systems and muscles, the more energy is in them as potential food. This is a metaphysical concept, but it has been proven over and over by nature and, ironically, by objective science—for science says that "energy cannot totally dissipate." This type of "energy" cannot be seen. Remember, energy never disappears; it merely changes form or goes from large to small, or liquid to gas. The energy from the Big Bang at the beginning of the universe is what keeps this planet moving and keeps us all alive. If we think of what we are eating in this way, a wild animal is much better than a cow, pig, or chicken which has been domesticated, which has lost three layers of energy—one from its domestication, one from the way these domesticated animals are forced to be raised in tight quarters (easier for slaughter), and one from how the animals are fed (not given free-range and pastured lives). We go from wild animal and wild food for the animal, to domesticating (altering wildlife), to feeding that sedentary animal cheap sacks of crappy grain (that we know is not natural to this earth), to enslaving them into a space less than the size of an average American freezer.

THE HUMAN PHYSIOLOGICAL CONSEQUENCES OF FOOD PRODUCTION

The *average* Upper-Palaeolithian (and to some extent the Neolithian) male was 6'1" tall, while the average female was 5'7" tall. They were almost always classically mesomorphic (muscular, wide, but lean), with an amazing balance of slow- and fast-twitch muscle fibers which allowed for both quick, explosive strength, and the ability to run long distances. This phenomenal athletic ability was without question the result of thousands of years of hunter-gatherer culture—exercising daily and eating *wild* (and sometimes raw) meat and *wild* roots, vegetables, nuts, fruits, and seeds.

With the advent of plant and animal domestication, the human skeleton started shrinking approximately three-fourths of an inch for each millennium that we moved forward (closer to the here and now). Only during the Middle Ages was the average European male a bit taller, and then those who came after those "dark ages," those direct descendants of the once super-athletic Upper Palaeolithians, were approximately 5'6" and had the physique of a modern-day couch potato (that wonderful, masculine, "pear-shaped" male). A total loss of eight inches in 9,000 years and a shape of a super-athlete reduced to a pear! How did this happen? The decrease in wild, dense animal protein, an increase in mutant grain consumption, an increase in saturated fat due to the higher levels found in sedentary, grain-fed, domesticated animals, and the steady loss of vigorous physical activity (by both the animals which we eat and our own physical activity) all contributed to this loss of stature (height and shape). This is not some kind of fiction story; rather, this is how we *devolved* away from being great physical specimens into sickly, helplessly addicted and pill-popping, neurotic, asymmetrical, fatty, and fast-food eating junkies. I am not talking about everyone, but think about how much you have to work out and "diet" just to get a glance from the opposite sex, never mind being healthy!

CONCLUSIONS ABOUT AGRARIANISM

Many very important conclusions can be drawn from studying these historical events pertaining to food production, which also had a huge bearing on the way we eat and live today, as well as how the world has been shaped culturally, religiously, and geopolitically.

1. The introduction of grains as a primary food source weakened the human physiology to a large degree. (Remember, these bad grains were "whole" grains, not the pulverized, refined flour from grains that many eat today). This is one of the many reasons I believe in eliminating all refined foods and, for most, all grains. This is also

Very Important

good enough evidence for me to choose to eat plenty of pure animals (meaning free-range, pastured, and not drugged), eggs (from "organic," pastured chickens), and wild fish protein, provided they are all clean of drugs, pollutants, and grain feed and are low in saturated fat. These animals can only be raised in a "free-range" type of way to have even a small chance of having that wild energy and low saturated fat that our great-ancestors found in the wild animals that they hunted down.

As a side note, the North American continent some 50,000–12,000 years ago was no different than the continent of Africa in the sense of what type of wild animals lived here. Lions, tigers, giraffes, zebras, elephants, and all of the exotic game which we automatically believe are uniquely indigenous to Africa all roamed the North American, and to some degree the South American, continents. Where did they all go, you ask? They were all hunted to extinction by our greatest ancestors, and when I say our "greatest ancestors," just imagine the sheer strength, speed, and power (not to mention the guts) it took to hunt down and kill, skin, and eat every part of a wild animal which could easily kill many men, had it not been for all of those aforementioned skills. Yes, the real world was cruel, and it was about survival.

The best way to eat today—in this world of drug-filled, poorly raised domesticated animals—is to buy freshly ground, free-range, pastured, non-antibiotic, and non-drugged chickens (and by 'drugged' I mean growth hormone, antibiotics, and/or steroids). I also eat eggs from similar chickens and *wild* salmon as sources of protein. Of course, I eat nothing made from grains—only vegetables, fruits, nuts, seeds, and roots such as potatoes, ginger, and so forth.

2. Agrarianism and food producing would lead us into our three modern nutritional dilemmas:

a) The pancreas is being overwhelmed with refined carbohydrates (pulverized flour products, which includes all pasta, rolls, bagels, pizza and breads, whether it says "whole wheat" or not), and our bodies are aging faster because of the increased insulin levels needed to store these refined forms of grains (and other man-made carbohydrates) as glucose. Increased insulin leads to insulin resistance, which leads to a host of problems such as diabetes, arterial sclerosis, and death (much more on this later).

b) We have become so reliant on food production that we are at the mercy of two powerful lobbying firms representing farmers who use antibiotics, steroids, and growth hormones to either fatten the beef or keep the animals from spreading germs and bacteria within their horribly confined living quarters before being slaughtered. Moreover, the secretary of agriculture pays (not directly—the treasury does that) some grain farmers to keep so much grain, store so much grain, ship so much overseas, and so forth. If you do not find a bit of conflict of interest in there, I am not sure you are reading me. Grains are a cheap way to feed the masses—all over the world!!

c) The *energy* of a domesticated plant such as wheat, or that of a sedentary cow, is weak and counter-evolutionary—even devolutionary. On top of that, we have been exposed to animal tissue which has been not only genetically altered but, in the past fifty years at least, chemically altered. There can be no doubt that eating these genetically and chemically altered species has not only changed our physiology, but it has also changed our "energy," resulting in that part of the day when everyone needs caffeine in order to "*make it through the next few hours.*" (Many people use cocaine, methamphetamines, crack, amphetamines, Sudafed, and even "health-food supplements" to stay awake or give them energy—this is a poor practice to get into).

Even though today Americans and Europeans are bigger and stronger than any time since the Neo-Paleolithic era, mostly because of the fact that we all eat adequate supplies of protein, the amount of body fat on a contemporary person has increased three-fold because of total caloric increase, especially in the form of high-glycemic carbohydrates, refined carbohydrates, and higher levels of saturated fat in livestock. The more refined and processed food we eat as post-modern humans, the further away from true evolutionary physiology and dynamic energy we will go. I have no doubt about this. All one has to do is follow the graph of cancers and type II diabetes. From what is known, both have steadily risen since the advent of the gristmill at the beginning of the Industrial Revolution, and that is only what we can plot with certainty.

It seems to me that there is an actual physiological and psychological change that takes place when eating food taken directly from a tree, the ground, or from animals which lived wild, as compared to food which has been made synthetically. What history teaches us—and what science tells us today—is what we should eat and how and why we age from what we eat. Let's look into this scientifically.

CHAPTER III

WHY AND HOW WE AGE: AN ORGANIC EXPLANATION

THE UNIVERSAL BIOLOGICAL
MARKERS OF AGING

First let us establish exactly what a biological marker is. Biological markers are measurable, quantifiable, and universal. They can be tracked throughout human history and observed over time. They cross all ethnic, racial, and gender barriers. For example, the fact that systolic blood pressure tends to rise as we age, regardless of ethnicity, race, or gender, is a biological marker.

There are four biological markers which *increase* with age and six which *decrease* with age.[8] (See graphic below.)

Markers Which Increase with Age	Markers Which Decrease with Age
insulin resistance	glucose intolerance
systolic blood pressure	aerobic capacity
percentage of body fat	muscle mass
lipid ratios	Strength
	temperature regulation
	immune function

---

8 Within the past few years, a cardiologist named Dr. Al Sears has been tracking, monitoring, X-raying, and documenting lung capacity with aerobic and anaerobic athletes. His conclusion is that doing resistance training is better for lung capacity than is aerobics. He believes this is also a biological marker of aging, but not everyone has agreed to this point on that, thus I have not used it here—despite the fact that his work is slowly gaining prominence. See "Notes" for more information.

AGE-RELATED BIOLOGICAL MARKERS

In contemplating on the chart on page 23, one can quickly see that there is an interesting correlation between what *increases* with age and what *decreases*. The increase in one's insulin resistance, for example, leads to a greater chance for developing glucose intolerance. As cells become *resistant to insulin*, there are *higher levels of glucose* remaining in the blood. Likewise, a person's decreased aerobic capacity means that the heart must work that much harder to the move the blood into outlying areas, thereby paving the way for chronic *high systolic blood pressure*. As more insulin is secreted due to high-glycemic carbohydrates and/or overeating, cells become more resistant and one begins to store higher levels of adipose tissue or *body fat*. This, in turn, *increases* LDL (low density lipoprotein) levels and almost simultaneously increases the chance for arterial sclerosis and other coronary problems. These conditions are of special concern for people who have a family history of heart disease. Further, the amount of body fat that people carry is directly related to how much insulin they produce and how little lean muscle mass they have. The lower one's percentage of *lean muscle mass,* the less support one's skeleton enjoys, and therefore a limiting of functionality will ultimately ensue. Limited functionality, in turn, gives way to a *loss of strength*, which then leads to a decrease in growth hormone production, the component needed for muscle building. Increased levels of stored body fat also slow the tissue repair process. If the tissue repair process takes too long, muscles risk atrophying from non-use, and lipid ratios will begin to rise. With a rise in lipid ratios, *temperature regulation* systems begin to fail, and the body's immune functions are ultimately compromised. Each of the body's other systems will begin to fail, too, and the negative aspects of the aging process become readily apparent.

Luckily, all of these aging processes are reversible—if you are willing to watch your diet and participate in a moderate workout program. Each of these biological markers is influenced by how and what we eat, how we use our bodies for exercise and/or motion, and to some degree, how well we regulate our emotions. Immortality remains out of the question, but careful attention to diet and exercise will help us to maintain our health longer and to live a more vital life.

From these observations, we can deduce that there are four known primary mechanisms which affect these biological markers. According to a theory postulated by Bernard Streheler in the late 1980s, an aging *mechanism* explains why we experience a loss in physiological function over time. This same mechanism must also explain why this loss is gradual and why the losses are intrinsic.

SCIENTIFIC THEORIES ON AGING

There are many schools of thought regarding the mechanisms of aging. One theory proposes that aging is programmed in our DNA. This theory suggests that there is a metaphorical clock ticking for each of us, and when the programmed hour arrives, you die. Russian aging expert Vladimir Dilman first proposed this theory, asserting that the internal "clock" could be found in the brain's hypothalamus, the home of the endocrine system, the part of the brain considered the "control central" for hormonal communication.

The hypothalamus is influenced by feedback loops that respond to hormonal levels. All of the body's physiological systems are affected by hormones; therefore, this theory not only makes good scientific sense, but it also gives us an opportunity to consider the possibility of a definite link between hormonal communication and aging. If this is true, we can assume that how we choose to eat and exercise can certainly affect our overall health and longevity, given that diet and exercise have such a profound effect on the endocrine system.

An alternative theory on aging, espoused by Robert Sapolsky of Stanford University, focuses on the glucocorticoid cascade mechanism. Sapolsky argues that, as levels of the corticosteroid cortisol are released by the adrenal glands during times of physical, emotional, or endocrine[9] stress, the body begins to store the cortisol, which over time leads to the death of neurons within the brain. As these neurons die or are damaged, the feedback message is also damaged, which leads to a release of even greater amounts of cortisol into the bloodstream. A catch-22 develops, and the autocrine[10] and endocrine systems fail. Death is not too far behind. As anyone who has ever taken any type of corticosteroid knows, it doesn't take these powerful hormones much time to affect nearly all aspects of the body.

Eicosonoid production (the underlying autocrine hormone that regulates not only the heart rate, but also the entire immune system) is also affected by the introduction of excess corticosteroids. Nevertheless, eicosonoids are, historically, a part of the oldest hormonal system of the body (the autocrine system). They are, as Dr. Barry Sears of "The Zone" diet plan likes to cali them, "*the molecular glue that holds all the body's systems together.*"

An extreme example of a cascading mechanistic failure brought on by hormone levels can be found in the life of the Pacific salmon. After swimming against heavy currents for several weeks, the salmon reaches its desired mating destination, only to mate and die within days. How and why, you might ask? The relentless struggle against the current leaves the salmon's body inundated with the stress hormone cortisol. Cortisol levels are too high, and all of the salmon's systems then fail. Elevated cortisol levels are responsible for all kinds of maladies in humans and animals alike, such as stroke, cancer, and heart disease. You must keep this in mind as you begin working out over long and frequent periods. Working out inherently subjects the body to stress, and stress produces cortisol; therefore, I have developed a way to train which is focused on short, intense workouts which also incorporate mild cardiovascular

---

9   Chronically high levels of insulin bring on endocrine stress.
10   The autocrine system regulates cell migration.

work, such as brisk walking, and mild, frequent stretching. The combination of these elements will help lower your levels of cortisol production.

Another mechanism of aging has been identified through DNA research focused on the tail-like fragments attached to the tips of chromosomes. These fragments are called *telomeres*. Each time a new cell division occurs, the telomere is shortened slightly. After so many divisions, the telomere is depleted, and the cell dies. Scientists have determined that, in order to fight the forces of aging, cell division should be kept to a minimum. How can we achieve this? Let us see.

The on/off process of DNA replication is controlled by the body's production of what are known as "growth factors." Insulin, which functions primarily as a storage hormone, is one of the most powerful growth factors of all. Bodybuilders who take insulin and growth factor-1, age anywhere from two to five times more quickly than normal, depending on how much sugar they eat and how much cortisol they produce. Moderate exercise, you will be pleased to learn, can offset the negative effects of insulin and growth factor production. A moderate level of exercise only produces the slightest amounts of cortisol. In addition, glucose uptake during exercise is not an insulin-driven event. That is to say, blood sugar and insulin levels both decrease and are normalized by regular, moderate exercise.

THE FINAL WORD ON INSULIN

The more insulin you produce, the more your cells are encouraged to grow. The more cell growth you experience, the more protein your body requires. The more protein you require, the more cell growth you will achieve, and therefore you will deplete an increasing number of telomeres. Therefore, we can conclude that there is a very fine line between producing enough insulin to store nutrients in cells and producing too much insulin to maintain regular health. In addition, excessive amounts of exercise will lead to excessive cell growth (division) and an unnecessary depletion of telomeres.

FREE RADICALS AND ANTIOXIDANTS

In the 1950s, Denham Harman developed an interesting theory on aging: the free radical concept of disease. Harman believed that aging was a consequence of an overproduction of *free radicals*—atoms or molecules with an unpaired electron.

The air which we breathe is, according to scientists, comprised of relatively inert gassy molecules. Unless the body extracts an electron from an oxygen atom (O2) to form a free radical, it cannot react with other molecules to maintain the constantly vigorous processes which control the body and give us life. Once the electron is extracted, an oxygen free radical forms, and aerobic life can begin. During the first 3 billion years on this planet, life was anaerobic; the photosynthetic process had not yet begun, and the single-celled microorganisms present on Earth did not require oxygen. With the emergence of photosynthetic organisms approximately 3.5 to 2.75 billion years ago, oxygen began accumulating in the atmosphere, and aerobic organisms developed to take advantage of this new oxygen-rich environment.

These early aerobic organisms devised ways to convert oxygen into water and, in turn, used the extraction process to create energy. Remember this, for this concept is very much tied into ATP[11] production and the forces which govern muscles during weight training and other short-term anaerobic exercises. The body constantly produces ATP to provide for short bursts of energy. To make this ATP, you must first produce an oxygen free radical. Under normal circumstances, a person only has enough ATP to last for about ten seconds before the body must make more—which requires more free radical production. This is why Burke's Law advocates efforts to increase your capacity to produce ATP. As ATP is used, lactic acid is released into the fatigued muscle, thus inhibiting its continued use. From a biological standpoint, training with weights in order to build muscle and increase strength should be done in short bursts of all-out effort, allowing just enough resting between sets for the body to make more ATP. Any other training method will not be as effective and borders on aerobic training, which does not build muscle or strength as effectively as anaerobic work. Remember, the body *must* produce ATP from free radicals; unfortunately, approximately 6 percent of all free radicals produced will escape to become "rogue" free radicals. Those which roam free remain unpaired and naturally begin looking for a mate. They seek out neighboring molecules in the body and attach themselves in an effort to become "whole." If this neighbor happens to be protein, DNA, or fat, this new molecule in turn becomes a new free radical.

The natural opponents of free radicals are antioxidants. Leading antioxidants include vitamins A, C, and E, selenium, and alpha lipoic acid. These vitamins are called antioxidants because they sacrifice themselves in an effort to stop this rogue free radical propagation, which, if left unchecked, will lead to the *oxidization* and death of cells. Vitamins don't, of course, stop aging or guarantee health, but they certainly do a great deal to help slow this natural degenerative process. An easy way to visualize the oxidization process is to think of a piece of metal which has been exposed to water and the elements. Rust develops, and small areas are destroyed. This is exactly what happens to cells when free radicals are made. Consequently, you should avoid overeating and over-exercising; this will reduce free radical formation and cell death.

---

11   ATP consists of adenosine—itself composed of an adenine ring and a ribose sugar—and three phosphate groups (triphosphate). The phosphoryl groups, starting with the group closest to the ribose, are referred to as the alpha (•), beta (•), and gamma (•) phosphates. ATP is highly soluble in water and is quite stable in solutions between pH 6.8–7.4, but it is rapidly hydrolysed at extreme pH. Consequently, ATP is best stored as an anhydrous salt.

If cellular defense enzymes and antioxidants, such as superoxide dimutase (SOD),[12] are not present or successfully made, the newly formed free radicals can cross-link with other free radicals to form *polymerized* products. Polymerized products can be a serious problem because they contribute to rapid cellular degeneration and aging.

Supplementing your diet with essential fatty acids such as omega-3 is vital for your health. These fats, however, are easily removed by oxygen free radicals, thus leaving behind a new free radical to react with oxygen to form a *peralkoxy free radical*. These new, more stable free radicals can inflict serious damage on cells as they seek out new electrons to strip. Once an essential fatty acid has been stripped and/or oxidized, it can no longer carry out its vital function of forming *eicosonoids*, the autocrine hormones which are the cellular foundation of the body's functions. When you supplement your diet with these essential fatty acids like omega-3, you are providing a valuable defense against the rogue free radicals that propel the aging process.

Returning for a moment to the so-called "rogue" free radicals—when a free radical attacks DNA molecule, a genetic mutation occurs, which, if unchecked, will be perpetuated during subsequent replication cycles. In other words, these damaged cells will not contain healthy DNA blueprints, and the cells will become prone to further mutation or attack, thus leading them to become cancerous.

As you can see, the more free radicals your body produces, the more rogue free radicals escape and attack the vital elements of your body. In descending order, food digestion, high levels of stress and the subsequent release of cortisol, and excessive amounts of exercise bring about free radical production. Digestion, by far, produces the most free radicals. Overeating, then, leads to an entirely avoidable increase in free radical production. Additionally, the more insulin-producing carbohydrates in your meals, the more energy digestion will require, and, of course, more free radicals will be produced.

Simply put, calories in food must be turned into a form of energy which the body can use; however, to form this fuel from food, it produces free radicals. Perhaps as much as 90 percent of all the free radicals you will make in your lifetime will come as a result of the digestive process. Later in this chapter, I will help you calculate how much food you should consume at each meal in order to guarantee adequate energy levels while still guarding against excessive free radical production.

After digestion, the primary way free radicals are generated is through the immune system. White blood cells are formed by free radicals in order to attack foreign invaders. Therefore, people with high or chronically low white blood cell counts often feel tired and rundown. Their immune systems are working overtime to produce white blood cells to fight off bacteria or a virus.

---

12   SOD is a "metal-containing antioxidant enzyme that reduces potentially harmful free radicals of oxygen formed during normal metabolic cell processes to oxygen and hydrogen peroxide." For more information, see the Medline Plus home page at the National Library of Medicine, http://www.nlm.nih.gov/medlineplus/mplusdictionary.html.

In addition to the three mechanisms of aging we have already discussed—increased cortisol, insulin, and free radical levels—there is one additional mechanism of aging remaining: the formation of *advanced glycocylated end-products* (AGEs).

AGEs are the most recently discovered of the mechanisms of aging and are responsible for the cross-linking of glucose (carbohydrates) and protein. AGEs have a very strong impact on aging and the development of degenerative illnesses. Anytime there are elevated levels of glucose in the bloodstream, it is likely that cross-linking will occur. That is to say, every time you overeat, especially if you have indulged in high-glycemic carbohydrates, cross-linking will occur, thereby doubling the speed of your aging process.

In addition to speeding the aging process, elevated glucose levels also result in damage to the glucose-sensitive region of the hypothalamus known as the *ventromedial nucleus*. This area of the hypothalamus is responsible for sending messages to the pancreas telling it when and how much insulin to secrete. Glucose-induced damage impairs this feedback system and results in the pancreas overproducing insulin. Insulin resistance is the natural consequence of this, as is the onset of type II diabetes.

Now that we have examined what speeds the aging process, let us try to figure out how to slow it down.

CHAPTER IV

HOW YOUR DIET AFFECTS THE BIOLOGICAL MARKERS OF AGING

As the previous chapter illustrated, there are four primary causes of aging:

1. Increased levels of cortisol
2. Excessive insulin levels
3. Excess free radicals
4. Excess glucose

This chapter will show you how best to regulate these four occurrences. First, let us turn our attention to excess insulin production, as a discussion of insulin levels will lead naturally to examinations of glucose and cortisol levels.

Despite many people's assumption that insulin has something to do with sugar (which it does), it is primarily a storage hormone. Insulin stores nutrients within cells. You must have adequate insulin levels in order to ensure proper feeding of your cells. Without it, they would suffer a rather quick death. However, too much insulin speeds aging and brings about death more quickly than almost any other biological process.

Excess insulin is produced when target cells no longer allow the insulin to store nutrients within the cell. When this happens, high glucose levels remain in the blood, and a feedback signal is sent to the hypothalamus, which in turn instructs the pancreas to secrete more insulin. At the same time, the affected cells begin to harden and become more rigid with each secretion of insulin, so the insulin begins to lose its ability to penetrate cells and store nutrients. Glucose levels remain high (potentially damaging brain cells and nerves) because penetration into cells is nearly impossible. In response to this, if the (insulin and other hormone) resistance becomes bad enough, the adrenal glands begin trying to regulate blood glucose with cortisol. The cells remain impenetrable, soon blocking the absorption of other hormones, and cell death begins.

The origins of age-related insulin resistance can be found by examining how our ancestors regulated their food consumption. Millions of years ago, humans did not eat "three square meals a day." Rather, starvation or deprivation conditions were the rule of the day. As a result, the pancreas was not called upon to secrete insulin several times per day as it is in modern Western culture. Insulin was able to store nutrients in cells, and excess calories went to adipose tissue, better known as body fat. This stored body fat was used later as much-needed fuel for hunting and, crucially, as an aid in the regulation of body temperature. It is also important to note here that the insulin produced by our ancestors was not designed to process the dense carbohydrates so commonly found in the refined foods many of us eat today.

Our bodies have an amazing ability to turn stored fats into fuel, provided the levels of glucose or insulin in the bloodstream are not high. For this reason alone, carbohydrates should be kept in balance with protein, since protein's pancreatic response, *glucagons*,[13] can counteract elevated levels of insulin in the blood. This is the notion upon which Barry Sears, founder of the popular "Zone" diet, has based his entire life's work. In my opinion, this is *the most* logical way to balance meals for effective hormonal communication and organ-to-cell communication. Having said this about how Barry has changed the way many of us think about food and hormones, I do not agree with Barry on every point in his first book. In his first book, he allowed one to use refined foods so long as their glucagon/insulin axis was balanced. I do not believe in eating any refined foods for a variety of reasons: they are like drugs and are hard to stop eating; they tend to be useless calories for the body; and the body can become "allergic" or sensitive to all refined foods, especially grains and flour made from grains. How would you like to be allergic to a refined food and have a hard time taking it out of your diet because you are addicted to it? This addiction is similar to drug addiction; however, the "detoxification" from refined food usually will only take two to four weeks. It will not be a pleasant month, but it is necessary for health and longevity.

CARBOHYDRATES

Insulin resistance, such as that which accompanies type II diabetes, occurs when, over a course of many years, a person who may or may not be predisposed—it really does not matter—takes in too many calories and/or too many high-glycemic carbohydrates at each meal. His or her cells become hardened and cannot absorb the micronutrients and macronutrients which insulin is designed to put into the cells.

High-glycemic carbohydrates[14] are those carbohydrates that induce the pancreas to secrete excessive amounts of insulin in order to store the condensed and relatively refined caloric content of the carbohydrate. They are termed "condensed" because the more a carbohydrate is refined, the more condensed it becomes, and the higher its glycemic factor. High glycemic factor carbohydrates require more

---

13   Glucagon is primarily a glucose mobilizer.
14   You can find the glycemic index on the Internet, in nutritional books at your local bookstore, or by going to http://www.glycemicindex.com/ or http://en.wikipedia.org/wiki/Glycemic_index.

insulin for storage. Three other nutritional factors also influence the glycemic index rankings of carbohydrates: (1) the amount of roughage in the carbohydrate (which influences its absorption rate and the rate of pancreatic insulin excretion); (2) the amount of fat taken in with the carbohydrate, which slows the absorption rate; and (3) the amount of protein absorbed, which influences glucagon and balances the insulin-related hormonal response of the pancreas. Each of these factors then slow insulin's release into the bloodstream and can help protect you against premature aging, hypoglycemia, type II diabetes, and the habitual storage of body fat. Be warned, however, that saturated fat— derived from domesticated animal products—can both increase insulin resistance and elevate LDL, or "bad" cholesterol. Most people with type II diabetes have insulin resistance as their main cause of high blood glucose.

High-glycemic carbohydrates are primarily found in foods made from refined grain products. A "refined" food is any food which has been altered from its original state. This even includes fruits dehydrated by the sun, such as raisins and other dried fruits. They are considered high-glycemic carbohydrates because their nutritional make-up is close if not equal to the simplicity and density of table sugar. Almost all breads and pastas, and all dehydrated foods, are also high on the glycemic index. You might wonder, "*Why are they there?*" These foods have high glycemic levels because the roughage and/or water naturally found within them have been removed, condensing them in such a way that the body overreacts to their refinement. Our bodies did not evolve by eating foods such as these, but rather our ancestors focused on killing wild game and gathering *whole wild foods*. The unnatural nature of a diet based on refined foods is borne out in the realization that approximately one third of the population of the United States is presently, or will become, diabetic. Additionally, one third of all Americans will die from heart disease which is directly related to their insulin output. Approximately 15 percent of Americans will develop cancers brought on by cortisol and insulin problems. We have the ability to organically live to be 120 years old. Most won't, because of these very problems which we have created with an abundance of refined food and high levels of stress with little knowledge of how to lower cortisol.

REFINED VS. "WHOLE" FOODS

Because they have been refined, foods which have been altered induce the pancreas to respond with an abundance of insulin, often times driving blood glucose levels down, in an attempt to store the dense molecules in cells and/or body fat. While some people can tolerate these foods relatively well due to a naturally buffered pancreatic response,[15] most people will eventually develop insulin-related

---

15   Those with this natural pancreatic "buffer" tend to be descended from the earliest groups of pre-agrarian humans. Those of Northern European ancestry, Native Americans, and most African-Americans, however, usually have not been blessed with this natural buffer. In my estimation after

problems. No matter whom you are, the more insulin you make, the greater and faster the potential for cellular deterioration and excessive free radical production.

Vegetables and fruits are generally considered low-glycemic carbohydrates because their high roughage content and low caloric levels keep the pancreatic response to a minimum. You should increase your intake of vegetables and (low calorie) fruits and restrict the grains and refined foods in your diet if you have any suspicion that you have insulin problems. If you suspect that you have insulin problems, but have not tested positive for them via standard sugar tests, you may still suffer from *reactive hypoglycemia*. If you are chronically fatigued, this may well be the source of your problems. Cut out all refined foods for three weeks and see if you improve. If so, you can assume you have this condition.

Given all this talk about the "bad" nature of carbohydrates, don't let yourself forget that you need some carbohydrates for proper brain and colon function. These carbohydrates are best supplied by roughage-rich fruits and vegetables. Minerals from the earth (where fruits and vegetables come) such as calcium and magnesium and the antioxidant vitamins A, C, E, and selenium, all at a microcellular level also help supply adequate amounts of slow-absorbing glucose for storage in muscles, the liver, and to aid in brain function.

The idea that fish is "brain food" is derived not only from its rich DHA and EPA content, but also because fish is an excellent source of protein, which makes glucagon and is used to mobilize stored glucose. This occurs when the pancreas is activated to secrete glucagon and then mobilizes glycogen stored in the liver and glucose stored in muscle tissues back into the bloodstream. In essence, the pancreas has three jobs: to secrete insulin when it senses carbohydrates coming in, to secrete glucagon when protein enters the body, and to store nutrients, hormones, and fats in the cells. When we ingest fish or healthy proteins, our brains work at their most efficient capacity and receive just the right amount of enzymes when blood glucose is stabilized and insulin is low. Ingesting too many carbohydrates and not enough protein, however, causes insulin to drive glucose levels down, and the body will not be able to make use of any stored glucose. This explains the "brain-dead" feeling that many people experience after large, carbohydrate-rich meals. Once again, you should not plan to eliminate carbohydrates altogether. That response is too far to the left. Rather, choose your carbohydrate sources wisely, and be sure to balance them with adequate levels of protein and fat in order to keep your glucose levels stable.

If your insulin levels are consistently high, cells will respond by becoming increasingly rigid, a state which hastens cell death. When we are young, cell membranes are fluid and soft, and insulin and other hormones such as human growth hormone, testosterone, and/or estrogen are easily able to penetrate the cell walls. Nutrients are easy to store within the cells, and therefore they are able to release energy as needed and ensure good tissue health. As we age, however, cell membranes

---

thirty years of training, plotting, and/testing clients, the number of those who are allergic or are food sensitive to grains is nearly 80-90 percent of the North American population.

naturally begin to harden (this is a direct result of the effect of insulin on their vital state over time), and communication between hormones and their target cells becomes increasingly difficult. Ironically, as this communication system fails, signals are sent to the hypothalamus indicating a need for even more insulin because glucose is not being stored properly.

If the insulin-absorbing system fails entirely, the hypothalamus will call for increased adrenal output, and the adrenal gland, in turn, will secrete cortisol in an attempt to drive down blood glucose levels. If this is allowed to take place, hypoglycemia or hyperinsulinemia will result. In extreme cases, adrenal failure may also occur. Do not allow yourself to reach this point! Hypoglycemia is, essentially, the first stage of type II diabetes. The bottom line is that the more insulin your body must produce, the faster you will age.

High glucose levels are deadly. Even though the brain has what is known as the "blood-brain barrier" to keep harmful substances out of the brain, glucose can still enter because of specific glucose-receptor sites. The glucose enters and then causes damage to the ventromedial nucleus (VMN) if levels are too high. These elevated glucose levels eventually lead to permanent nerve and tissue damage.

PROTEIN

Protein is the building block for all bodily tissues and is the foundation of the immune system. Not only is protein a building source, but it also has a stabilizing effect on glucose levels. Science has shown us that nitrogen levels, which indicate tissue repair and muscle growth (or the lack thereof), must be maintained at relatively moderate, stable levels throughout the day for optimum muscle hypertrophy and overall health. If these (nitrogen) levels drop sharply, tissue repair is either less effective or muscles begin to atrophy. The best way to maintain these vital levels is to ensure that you are consuming enough protein. As a rule, if you are a very active adult, you should take in at least 1 gram (professional athletes, 2 grams) of protein per pound of lean body weight every day. Find your ideal intake of low-glycemic carbohydrates by adding 1.25X your lean body mass for an average person who walks three times per week. For a person who trains with weights three times a week, this number should be 1.50, and for a professional athlete or semi-professional who does weight training three times a week and another sport or MMA (Mixed Martial Art) two to three times a week, this number should be 1.75 to 2.0 (remembering that the protein intake should be at least 2 grams per each pound of lean body weight for such an accomplished athlete).

This would mean, for instance, that an average physically active man weighing 200 pounds, with a body fat percentage of 10 percent, would require 180 grams of protein per day. Have your lean muscle mass calculated by a health professional to determine how many grams of protein your body requires. Take your servings of protein, add in calculated amounts of carbohydrates and monounsaturated fats, and divide them into four or five meals per day. Whenever possible, space the meals four hours apart for maximum nutrient absorption and the least amount of insulin response to your caloric intake.

PROTEIN SOURCES

Before you run out to the health food store to buy buckets of protein powder or charge to your meat market to buy yourself some fatty steaks, we need to review protein sources for a moment. Pre-modern cultures relied heavily upon wild game such as buffalo, wild deer, and elk for their protein sources. While game meat is naturally lean and free of the hormonal additives present in so much of our modern stock, it is not practical for us to swear off all but game meat in our search for healthy protein sources. Other good sources for protein are lean meats such as skinless chicken, turkey, the leanest beef, fish (the oilier the better), and eggs (without the yolks). Seek out poultry and beef which were raised organically and "free-range," (and/or "pastured) and not chained to a post or confined in one small area. These animals also should not have been fed steroids, antibiotics, or anything else devised to produce the fattest possible animals in the shortest amount of time.

Soy and other vegetable protein sources are acceptable too, but they are much less vital and supply fewer nutrients than meats do. It is my belief that vegetarianism is not the healthiest food choice one can make over the course of a lifetime. It is often difficult for vegetarians and vegans to maintain adequate levels of protein. A lack of protein will lead to caloric deficits; all too often, increased amounts of carbohydrates or saturated fats will end up filling this void. This is a double-whammy in terms of fat accumulation and increased insulin levels. We need look no further than our earlier example of the Upper-Paleolithic man to see that eating a diet rich in both meat and vegetables is our best way to maintain muscle mass into our later years and to take maximum advantage of our life span's potential.

As a final thought on protein, I would also caution you against eating fatty meats cooked over an open flame. Many recent studies have shown that open-flame cooking produces potentially carcinogenic enzymes from the meat as the saturated fat drips on the flames, and the smoke then sends off a highly carcinogenic group of molecules into the cooking meat.

FATS

Now that we have reviewed proteins and carbohydrates, we must take a look at fats. As previously mentioned, *saturated* fat, which is derived from animal sources, should be kept to an absolute minimum. Not only does saturated fat increase LDL cholesterol levels, it also contributes to insulin resistance. As a result of our modern domestication techniques of "fattening" our meat supplies, saturated fat levels have climbed far too high in both meat supplies and dairy products. *Monounsaturated* fats, those that are derived from certain nut plants and other vegetable sources, are much healthier than saturated fats. Monounsaturated fats should comprise the bulk of your fat intake. Olives and olive oil, some nuts such as almonds, avocados, and canola oil are all good examples of monounsaturated fats.

MEAL BALANCING

Presumably, you have by now calculated your lean body mass and protein requirements. The next step in developing your ideal nutritional plan is to calculate your ideal low-glycemic carbohydrate[16] intake requirements. To continue with our earlier example of a 200-pound man with 10 percent body fat (and thus a lean body mass and protein requirement of 180 grams per day), we would find that his daily carbohydrate requirement would be 225 grams, which should, of course, be eaten in conjunction with proteins and fats, never by themselves, and should be spread out over four or five small meals.

Finally, you will need to determine your daily monounsaturated fat requirements. Ideally, calories from monounsaturated fats should account for no more than 20 percent of your total caloric intake for the day. Again, based on these figures we have been using, our subject needs no more than three to four teaspoons of olive oil or canola oil per day. Saturated fats should be avoided whenever possible. In addition to monounsaturated fats, supplementing your diet with molecularly distilled fish oils is also very important. Four to eight grams daily should be sufficient. If you eat in this way, you will ensure that your autocrine (eicosonoid) system's hormonal communications are operating at maximum efficiency and, therefore, that your endocrine and paracrine hormones will work to their maximum potential. This, in turn, will increase natural growth hormone receptor sites in the body, slowly reversing cellular aging and modulating vascular problems such as high or low blood pressure.

A simple way to remember these portion recommendations while dining out would be to request a lean piece of protein approximately the size and thickness of the palm of your hand. Opening your hand and spreading your fingers out will give you an approximation of the amount of low-glycemic carbohydrates you should consume (mainly green vegetables). Finally, the size of your thumb will provide you a

---

16   For future reference, those carbohydrates under 60 on the glycemic index are primarily fruits and vegetables.

good estimate for calculating your monounsaturated fat allotment for the meal. For dessert, choose a piece of fruit rather than cake or ice cream.

Do not overeat at any meal, and do not eat fats, carbohydrates, or protein by themselves, as doing so will ultimately compromise the balance of hormone production. By eating frequent, smaller meals, you will keep your nitrogen levels high and therefore secrete more growth hormone, which, as you know, will help you to maintain muscle tissue longer as you age. Finally, by eating in this way, you will be able to keep your body's production of rogue free radicals to a minimum.

CHAPTER V

FOOD AND YOUR HORMONES

.

HOW FOOD INFLUENCES HORMONE PRODUCTION

As we have discussed, the autocrine system is the underlying hormonal system for all bodily functions because it controls the communication between the body's other two hormonal systems, the endocrine and paracrine. *Auto* comes from the Greek word *avro,* meaning self, by oneself, or independently. In endocrinology, autocrine hormones, or "first system" hormones, are often overlooked because of their unique ability to communicate on the cellular level; they do not rely on the bloodstream for communication. Because these messages are conveyed at the untraceable cellular level, they vanish in seconds. The more advanced endocrine and paracrine systems are paid a great deal more attention by doctors and scientists because they leave a trail in the bloodstream. Eicosonoids control all functions on the cellular level and are the hormones that are most influenced by which foods you choose. How they are combined, in turn, affects glucagon and insulin production. Glucagon and insulin are autocrine hormones. This is a key point: what we eat affects these hormones tremendously.

To better understand this, we must go back to a time when single-cell organisms existed. In single-cell organisms, communication was only necessary across the cell itself, and simple chemical signals developed to speed this process. As time passed and organisms started becoming more complex, two or more cells needed to communicate. This very basic intercellular system works relatively well when all of the cells in question are of the same sort, but if there are too many cells in need of the information, the process becomes very slow. The nervous system developed when the early cell-to-cell communication systems no longer proved adequate for message delivery. The advent of nerves provided a speedy, remote way for organisms to communicate within themselves. Hormones were the next logical step in this communicative process. They enabled cells to develop and react to messages more quickly and accurately than ever before.

Finally, after the development of the nervous system and hormones, the endocrine system emerged. It uses the bloodstream to pass messages and employs the nervous system as its "feedback loop." Both the paracrine and endocrine hormonal systems are directly influenced in their signals, feedback, and so-called "second messengers," the autocrine hormones, eicosonoids. The better one's autocrine hormonal health (cell-to-cell communication), the more freely the other two more complex hormonal systems will work.

TEN NUTRITIONAL RULES FOR LONGEVITY AND BUILDING MUSCLE MASS

1. Eat four to six small meals per day, in accordance with the ratios given in this book and in *The Zone*, by Barry Sears. Choose a diet comprised mostly of vegetables and fruits, and rely on them to be your primary sources for carbohydrates. Stay away from a lot of bread and pasta-laden meals. Unlike the plan outlined in *The Zone*, I do not recommend eating any refined food.
2. Eat lean meats, fish, eggs, and whey protein powder for protein sources.
3. Design a meal program that is comparable to those figures given in the protein section. Your protein intake should be based on 1 gram per pound of lean body mass.
4. Eat primarily low-glycemic carbohydrates. A glycemic index can be found on the Internet.
5. For fats, seek out and consume mostly monounsaturated fats, such as some nuts, avocados, olives, olive oil, canola oil, and so forth. Try to keep saturated fats to a minimum. (All animal products contain saturated fat, as do cashews and peanuts).
6. Supplement your diet with EPA fish oil capsules.
7. Don't overeat, even if you missed a meal earlier in the day. Organize each meal this way: Protein portions should be the size and thickness of the palm of your hand. Low-glycemic carbohydrates should take up three times as much space as the protein on your plate. Fats should equal approximately the size of your thumb, or slightly more.
8. Supplement your diet with the antioxidants and minerals listed in the nutritional section of this book and any others that your nutritionist or other health practitioner might recommend. Stay away from so-called "growth supplements."
9. Drink plenty of water throughout the day; however, do not force yourself to drink a lot of water. Where this comes from, I have no idea. All one has to do is go out into nature and watch a deer for a day (if you can)—it will just sip a bit of water from a cool brook every so often. It is foolish to drink a lot of water unless you are thirsty and/or exercising.
10. Stick with it! Discipline is a vital part of your health and fitness plan.

CHAPTER VI

GRAINS: HOW BAD ARE THEY?

I am not the only person thinking about and researching grains. From the following sources comes some interesting observations.

Brought to you by Mark's Daily Apple.[17]

"Grains. Every day we're bombarded with them and their myriad of associations in American (and much of Western) culture: Wilford Brimley, Uncle Ben, the Sunbeam girl, the latest Wheaties athlete, a pastrami on rye, spaghetti dinners, buns for barbeque, corn on the cob, donuts, birthday cake, apple pie, amber waves of grain…. Gee, am I missing anything? Of course. So much, in fact, that it could, and usually does, take up the majority of supermarket square footage. (Not to mention those government farm subsidies, but that's another post). Yes, grains are solidly etched into our modern Western psyche, just not so much into our physiology. When I say humans didn't evolve eating grains, I mean our digestive processes didn't evolve to maximize the effectiveness of grain consumption. Just because you can tolerate grains to a certain degree, as just about all of us can (thanks to those earlier folks hitting the end of the genetic line), doesn't mean your body was designed for them or that they're truly healthy for you. We're not talking about what will allow you to hobble along. We're talking about the foods that offer effective and efficient digestion and nutrient absorption in the body. And that's all about evolutionary design."

Mark is right, as I have said throughout this book, grains are terrible on the body and many other systems; however, there are a few more key points to bring up here.

For instance, *gluten* and *lectins*, are both initiators of digestive chaos, you might say. Gluten, the large, water-soluble protein that creates the elasticity in dough, is found in most common grains like wheat, rye and barley (and believe it or not, it is the primary glue in wallpaper paste).

17   The entire philosophy can be found online at http://stanford.wellsphere.com/healthy-eating-article/the-definitive-guide-to-grains/11919.

Researchers now believe that a third of us are likely gluten intolerant/, or gluten-sensitive[18]. Over time, those who are gluten intolerant can develop a dismal array of medical conditions: slowly progressive arthritis, dermatitis, joint pain, reproductive problems, acid reflux, and other digestive conditions, autoimmune disorders such as Lupus and even MS, and Celiac disease. This still doesn't mean that the rest of the population is not experiencing some milder negative effect which simply doesn't manifest itself so obviously—because almost everyone has some negative effect from gluten.

Lectins are mild, natural toxins that aren't limited to just grains, but seem to be found in especially high levels in most common grain varieties—such as wheat and barely. These Lectins are one more reason to believe that grains just aren't worth all the trouble which comes with them. Lectins, researchers have found, inhibit the natural repair system of the GI tract, potentially leaving the rest of the body open to the impact of errant, wandering (i.e., unwanted) material from the digestive system, especially when these lectins "unlock" barriers to entry and allow larger undigested protein molecules into the bloodstream. This breach can initiate all kinds of immune-related havoc and is thought to be related to the development of autoimmune disorders. Some people are more sensitive to the damage of lectins than others, as in the case with gluten.

GRAINS AND THE BRAIN

Evolution is surely an interactive process. In the early stages of our evolution, it was all about strength, power, the senses and eventually wisdom. Today, those of us who learn quickly and well are more likely to survive, thrive, and reproduce. Learning capacities then, are factors in the survival of our genes. Research is now revealing that cereal grains, along with breads, pastas and other allergenic and highly glycemic foods, pose a serious threat to our sustained ability to learn. These foods have been shown to interfere with almost any stage of the learning process, impeding our attempts to focus our attention, observe, ponder, remember, understand, and apply that understanding. Grains can alter learning capacities in four specific ways: as sequels of untreated celiac disease; through an immune sensitivity to gluten; through dietary displacement of other nutrients, and through the impact of grain on blood sugar/insulin levels. (Mothers and fathers, here is the "truth" about what your children are going through if they are eating anything made from grains—such as almost all cereals). All of a sudden, in this new millennia, every other child has either ADD or ADHD! Additionally, how is it possible that autism used to occur, just a few decades ago, in one out of 160,000 and now that figure is one in 160?

---

18   To repeat, personally, I believe that this number is eighty to ninety percent of the people on earth.

This is appalling! Recently, many parents have banded together in a fight against pharmaceutical companies who make vaccinations for children—believing all along that the mercury in those vaccines had turned their child into an autistic child. My honest belief is that sugary, grain-based, refined cereals are at the forefront of suspects for that which is causing the cases of autism to go up so dramatically.

There are many reports of learning problems in association with untreated celiac disease. A majority of children with celiac disease display the signs and symptoms of Attention Deficit Disorder (ADD/ADHD), a range of learning difficulties and developmental delays. Many of the same problems are found more frequently among those with gluten sensitivity, a condition signaled by immune reactions against this most common element of the modern diet. Grain consumption can also cause specific nutrient deficiencies that are known to play an important role in learning. Grains can also cause problems with blood sugar/insulin levels, resulting in reduced capacities for learning. Furthermore, foods derived from grain are an important element in the current epidemic of hypoglycemia, obesity, and Type 2 diabetes. Our growing understanding of the biological impact of cereal grain consumption must move educators to challenge current dietary trends.

Part of our improved understanding comes from new testing protocols which are revealing that celiac sprue afflicts close to 10 percent of the general population. It is widespread and appears to occur more frequently among populations which have experienced relatively shorter periods of exposure to these grains. The importance of this newly recognized high frequency of celiac disease becomes obvious when we examine the impact it has on learning and behavior.

Research has identified ADHD in 66—70 percent of children with untreated celiac disease, which resolves on a gluten-free diet, and returns with a gluten challenge. Several investigators have connected particular patterns of reduced blood flow to specific parts of the brain in ADHD. Other reports have connected untreated celiac disease with similarly abnormal blood flow patterns in the brain. One might be able to dismiss such reports if viewed in isolation, but the increased rates of learning disabilities among celiac patients, and the increased rates of celiac disease among those with learning disabilities leave little to the imagination. Further, there is one report of gluten-induced aphasia (a condition characterized by the loss of speech ability) that resolved after diagnosis and institution of a gluten-free diet. Still other investigations suggest a causal link between the partial digests of gluten (opioid peptides) and a variety of problems with learning, attention, and development.

Gluten sensitivity, afflicting close to 15 percent of the general population, is an immune reaction to one or more proteins found in grains. When a person's immune system has developed antibodies against any of these proteins, undigested and partly digested food particles have been allowed to enter the bloodstream. The leakage of food proteins through the intestinal wall signals a failure of the protective, mucosal lining of the gastrointestinal tract, as is consistently found in untreated celiac disease. (This is called "Leaky Gut Syndrome"). Many of the same health and learning problems which are found in celiac disease are significantly over-represented among those with gluten sensitivity for the very good reason that many of the same proteins are being leaked into the blood of those with gluten sensitivity.

Our cultural obeisance to grains is at odds with the remains of ancient humans. Archaeologists have long recognized that grains (were) and still are a starvation food—one for which we are not well suited. Grains result in consistent signs of disease and malnourishment in every locale and epoch associated with human adoption of grain cultivation.

Grains are a poverty food. As we increase our grain consumption, we cause deficiencies in other nutrients by overwhelming the absorptive and transport mechanisms at work in our intestines. For instance, diets dominated by grains have been shown to induce iron deficiency—a condition that is widely recognized as causing learning disabilities. This should not be surprising since iron is the carrier used to distribute oxygen throughout our bodies, including various regions of our brains. There is little room to dispute the hazards to learning posed by reductions in oxygen supply to the brain. Iron deficiency reduces available oxygen in the brain, revealing yet another dimension of gluten grains as mediators of learning difficulties.

In addition, the impact of grain consumption on our blood sugar levels is yet another facet of its contribution to learning problems. We evolved as hunter-gatherers, eating meats, and carbohydrates in the form of fruits, vegetables, and seeds. Refined sugars were a rare treat wrested from bees with some difficulty. At best, it was a rare treat for our pre-historic ancestors.

Today, with unprecedented agricultural/industrial production of refined sugars along with cultivation and milling of grain flours, these products have become very cheap and available, particularly over the last fifty years. During that time, we have added enormous quantities of grain-derived starches to the overwhelming quantities of sugar we consume. The result of this escalating dietary trend may be observed in the current epidemic rates of type II diabetes, hypoglycemia, obesity, and cardiovascular disease. In the classroom, we see these trends manifest in students' mood swings, behavioral disorders (fluctuating between extreme lethargy and hyperactivity), chronic depression, forgetfulness, and muddled thinking—all of which reflects the inordinate, counter-evolutionary burden placed on many homeostatic systems of the body, particularly those related to blood sugar regulation.

The pancreas has many functions. One important activity of the pancreas is to stabilize blood sugar levels. When blood sugar is not well regulated, learning is impaired. The pancreas secretes carefully monitored quantities of glucagon and insulin. The pancreas responds to the presence of proteins, sugar, and starch in the digestive tract by producing insulin. It produces glucagon in response to protein. The balanced presence of both of these hormones in the bloodstream is critical to learning because they regulate the transport of nutrients into cells. Too little or too much insulin can cause blood sugar levels go out of control inducing a wide range of symptoms.

Today, when the insulin/glucagon balance goes awry, it is frequently due to insulin overproduction in a diet dominated by sugars and starches. This overproduction is caused by chronic consumption of highly glycemic foods[19]. The resulting elevated levels of insulin cause rapid movement of nutrients into cells, either for storage as fat, or to be burned as energy, causing increased activity levels, "hot spells," sweating, increased heart rate, etc. This energized stage requires a constant supply of sugars and starches to be maintained. Otherwise, it is soon followed by bouts of lethargy, light-headedness, tremors, and weakness, which are all signs of hypoglycemia or very low blood sugar levels.

Despite having stored much of the blood sugars as fats, there is insufficient glucagon to facilitate its use for energy. As this condition progresses, and as blood sugar levels plummet, periods of irrational anger and/or confusion often result. These moods often result from adrenaline secreted to avoid a loss of consciousness due to low blood sugar levels. The next step in the progression, in the absence of appropriate nutritional intervention, is lapsing into a coma.

In the short term, the answer to these fluctuations is more frequent consumption of sugars/starches. However, the long-term result of such an approach is either a state of insulin resistance, where more and more insulin is required to do the same task, or a state of pancreatic insufficiency, where the pancreas is simply unable to keep pace with the demand for insulin. In either case, once this stage is reached, the individual may be diagnosed with type II diabetes. This disease has so increased among North Americans, particularly among children, that an autoimmune form of diabetes, previously called juvenile onset, had to be renamed to "Type I diabetes".

By now, it will not surprise the reader to learn that Type I diabetes has also been shown to be significantly associated with gluten. Research reveals that there is considerable overlap between celiac disease and Type I diabetes. About 8 percent of celiacs also have Type I diabetes, and 5-11 of Type I diabetics have celiac disease. Further, Scott Frazer et al. have repeatedly shown, in animal studies, a causal, dose-dependent relationship between type I diabetes and gluten.

The growing reaction against gluten and other allergenic foods should not be confused with the several dietary fads of the 20th Century. The vegetarian perspective ignores the vitamin deficiencies which result from a strict vegetarian diet. The low-fat craze is another fad which has mesmerized the industrialized world for the last 30–40 years[20]. Fortunately, this perspective has recently come under scrutiny. Despite having served as the driving force behind most physicians'

---

19   A new and updated Glycemic Index can be found at: http://www.mendosa.com/gilists.htm
20   After one famous scientific study done about heart health and fats, (Study done in Helsinki) in the 1960's, Americans began taking *all* fats from their diet in response to the study that showed how "high cholesterol" can and will cause heart problems, even death. Naturally, taking out all fats caused more heart-deaths from not having enough "good cholesterol" than when people were eating all types of fats. The answer is to eat "good fats" such as monounsaturated fats. Our culture is one of extremes and we have to begin to realize that most of nutrition and medicine lie in the gray areas of the body— those which are not so simply understood, nor found, nor "cured" with an extreme solution.

dietary recommendations during the last several decades, the low fat dictum is overwhelmingly being discredited by research reported in peer-reviewed publications.

Recognition and avoidance of allergenic and highly glycemic foods is a completely new trend which is based on scientific research and evidence. It reflects an improved understanding of the function of the gastrointestinal tract, the endocrine system, and particularly the pancreas and the immune system. Past dietary fads are consistently deficient in important nutrients which are necessary to our good health and survival. Furthermore, they frequently contain substances which are harmful to us, such as the phytates which are abundantly present in whole grain foods, and interfere with absorption of many minerals.

It is increasingly clear that grains, especially those that contain gluten, are contraindicated for human learning. The evidence is overwhelming. The mandate of eating to learn is learning to eat as our ancestors did.

1. Gluten is the general name used to describe proteins found in wheat and other cereal grains. Gluten is the sticky, elastic component of grains, essential for breads and baking. Any flour made from the starchy endosperm of grains contains proteins which are potentially problematic to the person with a gluten allergy.
2. Gluten is a mixture of proteins classified into two groups, the prolamines and the glutelins. The prolamine, gliadin, seems to be a major problem in celiac disease; anti-gliadin antibodies are found in the serum and in circulating immune complexes associated with this disease.
3. Wheat, barley, rye, and oats have been excluded from "gluten-free diets." Most evidence implicates wheat as the main problem food. Bread is the most desired wheat product and is, unfortunately, the hardest food to duplicate with non-grain flours.
4. Recent studies suggest that oats may not be as problematic as wheat. Both the type and the amount of the gluten proteins decide the kind of reaction which is likely to occur.
5. Immune responses to gluten, the proteins found in cereal grains, are a common cause of an impressive number of diseases. The remarkable fact is that eating "normal," often-recommended foods can be hazardous to your health. Celiac is the best defined gluten disease.
6. The classic presentation of celiac disease is chronic diarrhea, with abdominal bloating, sometimes pain, weight loss, iron deficiency, and other evidence of nutrient malabsorption. Celiac disease is immune-mediated and should be described as gluten allergy.
7. People who are diagnosed with celiac disease often feel like outcasts and resent the hard work of avoiding gluten. We have taken the opposite

approach and ask a much larger group of people to exclude gluten along with other popular foods as a routine measure of restoring health.

8. A list of diseases which occur with increased frequency in celiac patients resembles the list of disorders reviewed under our descriptions of delayed pattern food allergy. These diseases include diabetes, thyroid disease, anemia, rheumatoid arthritis, sacroileitis, sarcoidosis, vasculitis, inflammatory lung disease, eye inflammation, cerebellar ataxia, and schizophrenia. These and other immune-mediated diseases can be linked to gluten ingestion. These associations suggest that people with a tendency to immune hypersensitivity diseases are vulnerable to food antigens which can cause systemic autoimmune disease.

Gluten Intolerance can be diagnosed at any age and can be called a variety of names: celiac sprue, gluten-sensitive enteropathy, nontropical sprue, celiac disease, idiopathic steatorrhea or malabsorption syndrome. Celia sprue is a genetic, inheritable immunologic disease which interferes with the digestion process. The disease may affect as many as 10 times more people than originally thought, due to the fact that it can take up to 10 years to diagnose. It is estimated 1 in 133 people in the U.S. may be affected with intolerance to the gluten in wheat, and go undiagnosed. Gluten is the structure that holds the gas in bread to give it a light, airy texture. Gluten is a protein found in varying amounts in wheat, rye, barley, and perhaps oats. Foods which induce rhinitis, sinusitis, bronchitis, asthma, intestinal cramps, diarrhea, hives, angioedema, eczema, and migraines are said to be "allergenic" in certain individuals. Approximately 1.5 percent of adults and 5 to 8 percent of children, who usually outgrow them, suffer from food allergies.

Food allergies involve the immune system, with most allergic reactions occurring within 2 hours. Reactions to an allergen may also occur within seconds or take as long as 24 hours. According to the Food Allergy and Anaphylaxis Network, milk, egg, peanut, tree nut, fish, shellfish, soy, and wheat are the most common foods to cause allergic reaction.

Food intolerances may also cause adverse reactions and symptoms may be similar to food allergies. The key difference between a food allergy and food intolerance is that a food intolerance does not trigger the immune system. Since celiac sprue, wheat allergy and wheat intolerance are different diagnoses, treatment may be different. For example, some people with wheat allergies are not gluten intolerant and can eat rye, barley, and oats.

SYMPTOMS OF GLUTEN INTOLERANCE

The most common symptoms of gluten intolerance include cramps, diarrhea, growth failure in children, loss of appetite and menstrual irregularities.

The ability of the small intestine to absorb fat is affected and thus fat-soluble vitamin absorption is reduced. (Vitamins A and E to name the most important that are "fat soluable.")

Because carbohydrate and protein absorption is also affected, malnutrition can result if not treated. Children are especially vulnerable because of their growth needs. If treated through a gluten-free diet, teenagers may seem to "out-grow" the symptoms; however, celiac sprue still exists and the need to eliminate gluten from their diet is for life.

Doctors can biopsy the small intestine to diagnose celiac sprue. If eliminating all gliadin from the diet relieves the symptoms, the diagnosis is conclusive.

 A wheat "allergy" may manifest itself in a variety of symptoms including breathing disorders, skin rashes, cramps, and migraine headaches. (If you suspect; go to your Physician ASAP.)

CHAPTER VII

WHAT IS A MODERN-DAY PALEODIET?

It all began not that long ago when a gastroenterologist named Walter L. Voegtlin was one of the first to suggest that following a diet similar to that of the Paleolithic era would improve a person's health. (Naturally, I have read his book).

In 1975, when I was meeting Arnold Schwarzenegger for the first time[21], GI specialist Voegtlin published a book in which he argued that humans are carnivorous animals and that the ancestral Paleolithic diet was that of a carnivore—chiefly fats and protein with only small amounts of carbohydrates.[22] His dietary prescriptions were based on his own medical treatments of various digestive problems, namely colitis, Crohn's disease, irritable bowel syndrome, and indigestion.

In 1985, a decade after meeting Arnold, I won the Mr. Empire State bodybuilding contest in NYC and went on to take third place in the AAU (Jr.) Mr. Universe. That same year, Melvin Konner and S. Boyd Eaton, an associate clinical professor of radiology and an adjunct associate professor of anthropology at Emory University, published a key paper on Paleolithic nutrition in the *New England Journal of Medicine*. Their paper allowed this dietary concept to gain mainstream medical recognition. Three years later, S. Boyd Eaton, Marjorie Shostak, and Melvin Konner published a book about this nutritional approach, which was based on achieving the same proportions of nutrients (fat, protein, and carbohydrates, as well as vitamins and minerals) as were present in the diets of late Paleolithic people, not on excluding foods that were not available before the development of agriculture. As such, this

---

21   The only reason that I bring this up is to allow you a snapshot of what was happening in the world at that time—both to me, Arnold, and these people, who I would call, brilliantly ahead of their time. This and how important it was for me to have met Arnold at such a young age would influence me even more that I had made the right decision to become a bodybuilder (and then an actor—do you think Arnold had an impact on my life?)

22   This is where my way of eating and a paleodiet differ. I believe that we need plenty of vegetables and fruits, with far *less* fat than that of a paleodiet. Nevertheless, he was the first doctor/scientist to start down this path in modern times.

nutritional approach included skimmed milk, whole grain bread,[23] brown rice, and potatoes prepared without fat, on the premise that such foods have the same nutritional properties as Paleolithic foods. In 1989, these authors published a second book on Paleolithic nutrition.

Since the end of the 1990s, a number of medical doctors and nutritionists have advocated a return to a so-called Paleolithic (pre-agricultural) diet, as I have already mentioned. Proponents of this nutritional approach have published books and created Web sites to promote their dietary prescriptions. They have synthesized diets from commonly available modern foods which would emulate the nutritional characteristics of the ancient Paleolithic diet, some allowing specific foods which would have been unavailable to pre-agricultural peoples, such as certain processed oils and beverages.

[The Paleolithic diet is a modern dietary regimen which seeks to mimic the diet of pre-agricultural hunter-gatherers, one which corresponds to what was available in any of the ecological niches of Paleolithic humans. Based upon commonly available modern foods, it includes cultivated plants and domesticated animal meat as an alternative to the wild sources of the original pre-agricultural diet. The ancestral human diet is inferred from historical and ethnographic studies of modern-day hunter-gatherers as well as archaeological finds and anthropological evidence.

The Paleolithic diet consists of foods which can be hunted and fished, such as meat, fowl, and seafood, as well as foods which can be gathered, such as eggs, insects, fruit, nuts, seeds, vegetables, mushrooms, herbs, and spices. Practitioners are advised to eat only the leanest cuts of meat, free of food additives, preferably wild game meats and grass-fed beef since they contain relatively high levels of omega-3 fats, compared with grain-fed domestic meats. Food groups which were rarely or never consumed by humans before the Neolithic (agricultural) revolution are excluded from the diet, mainly grains, legumes (for example, peanuts), dairy products, salt, refined sugar, and processed oils, although some advocates consider the use of oils with low omega-6/omega-3 ratios, such as olive oil and canola oil, to be healthy and advisable. Practitioners are permitted to drink primarily water, and some advocates recommend tea as a healthful drink, but alcoholic and fermented beverages are restricted from the diet. Furthermore, eating a wide variety of plant foods is recommended to avoid high intakes of potentially harmful bioactive substances, such as goitrogens, which are present in certain roots, vegetables, and seeds. Unlike raw food diets, the Paleolithic diet does not limit the consumption of cooked foods. Cooking is widely accepted to have been practiced at least 250,000 years ago, in the early Middle Paleolithic.)

According to certain proponents of the (Upper) Paleolithic diet, practitioners should derive about 56–65 percent of their food energy from animal foods and 36–45 percent from plant foods. They recommend a diet high in protein (19–35%

23   This is where they stray from my ideologies—milk and wheat have been shown repeatedly to cause allergies and food sensitivities. Lactose intolerance in North America is on the rise.

energy) and relatively low in carbohydrates (22–40% energy), with a fat intake (28–58% energy) similar to or higher than that found in Western diets[24]. Furthermore, some proponents exclude from the diet, foods which exhibit high glycemic indices, such as potatoes.[25] Staffan Lindeberg, an associate professor in the Department of Medicine at the University of Lund, advocates a Paleolithic diet, but does not recommend any particular proportions of plant, versus meat or macronutrient ratios. According to Lindeberg, calcium supplementation may be considered when the intake of green leafy vegetables and other dietary sources of calcium is limited.

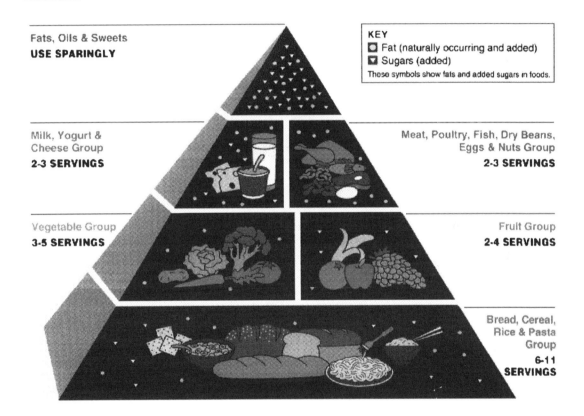

The USDA's Food Pyramid (above[26]) shows the food groups and the relative proportions of food consumed in the United States today, with grains and cereals at the base of the pyramid. The way my pyramid would be is vegetables on the bottom, protein from lean meats and fish, some fruits just below protein, nuts, seeds and berries (cherries) on top—that is it. The rest is killing all of us for various reasons.

---

24   Again, the importance of using the term "good fats" cannot be stressed enough. Good fats are as vital to heart health and hormonal stability as is protein. It is saturated fat that you want to stay away from.

25   I believe potatoes are fine to eat, but only on occasion.

26   Food Pyramid and other information in this section come from "Wikipedia."

very Important

According to S. Boyd Eaton, "*we are the heirs of inherited characteristics accrued over millions of years; the vast majority of our biochemistry and physiology are tuned to life conditions that existed prior to the advent of agriculture some 10,000 years ago. Genetically our bodies are virtually the same as they were at the end of the Paleolithic Era some 20,000 years ago.*"

As stated, (Upper)-Paleolithic nutrition has its roots in evolutionary biology and rests on the principles of evolutionary medicine. The reasoning underlying this nutritional approach is that natural selection had sufficient time to genetically adapt the metabolism and physiology of Paleolithic humans to the varying dietary conditions of that era. However, in the 10,000 years since the invention of agriculture and animal domestication and its consequent major change in the human diet, natural selection has had too little time to make the optimal genetic adaptations to the new diet.[27] Physiological and metabolic maladaptations result from the suboptimal genetic adaptations to the contemporary human diet, which in turn contribute to many of the so-called diseases of civilization.

Based on the subsistence patterns and biomarkers of hunter-gatherers studied in the last century, many people argue that modern humans are well adapted to the diet of their Paleolithic ancestor. The diet of modern hunter-gatherer groups is believed to be representative of patterns for humans of 50 to 25 thousand years ago. Individuals from these and other technologically primitive societies, including those individuals who reach the age of 60 or beyond, seem to be largely free of the signs and symptoms of chronic disease (such as obesity, high blood pressure, non-obstructive coronary atherosclerosis, and insulin resistance) which universally afflict the elderly in western societies (with the exception of osteoarthritis, which afflicts both populations). Moreover, when these people adopt western diets, their health declines and they begin to exhibit signs and symptoms of the "diseases of civilization." In one clinical study, stroke and ischaemic heart disease appeared to be absent in a population living on the island of Kitava, in Papua, New Guinea, where a subsistence lifestyle, uninfluenced by western dietary habits, was still maintained.

The results of initial prospective medical studies on the Paleolithic diet have shown positive health outcomes. The first animal experiment on a Paleolithic diet suggested that this diet, as compared with a cereal-based diet, conferred higher insulin sensitivity, lower C-reactive protein and lower blood pressure in domestic pigs. In the first controlled human trial on a Paleolithic diet, researchers found that the diet improved glucose tolerance more than a Mediterranean diet in individuals with ischaemic heart disease. Subsequently, a short-term intervention with the diet

---

27 As I said earlier in the book, it makes no difference as far as genetic adaptations because our organs cannot change any longer. I learned this during my master's program. Professor Chandler Steiner, who I speak of highly in the "Acknowledgements" area, showed me how any other adaptation to our body would be impossible at this stage, and anything other than that fact would be called "cultural Darwinism," meaning that culture cannot change organs, it can only change what we eat, do, believe and create.

in healthy volunteers showed some favorable effects on cardiovascular risk factors. Regarding this medical trial, the NHS Knowledge Service stated that there are several limitations to the study and that *"readers should not draw too many conclusions from it."* Two clinical trials designed to test various physiological effects of the Paleolithic diet are currently underway, and the results of two completed trials have not yet been reported.

With the advent of agriculture and the beginning of animal domestication roughly 10,000 years ago, during the Neolithic Revolution, humans started consuming large amounts of dairy products, beans, cereals, alcohol, salt and fatty domestic meats. In the late 18th and early 19th centuries C.E., the Industrial revolution led to the large scale development of mechanized food processing techniques and intensive livestock farming methods which enabled the production of refined cereals, refined sugars and refined vegetable oils, as well as fattier domestic meats, which have become major components of Western diets. Such food staples have fundamentally altered several key nutritional characteristics of the human diet since the Paleolithic Era, and these dietary compositional changes have been implicated as risk factors in the pathogenesis of many of the so-called "diseases of civilization[28]" and other chronic illnesses which are widely prevalent in Western societies, including obesity, cardiovascular disease, diabetes, osteoporosis, autoimmune-related diseases, certain cancers, myopia and acne, as well as many diseases related to vitamin and mineral deficiencies.

According to Cordain et al., the food staples and food-processing procedures introduced during the Neolithic and Industrial eras have fundamentally altered seven crucial nutritional characteristics of the ancestral human diet, which serve to inhibit the development of the diseases of affluence in modern-day hunter-gatherers, namely glycemic load, fatty acid composition, macronutrient composition, micronutrient density, acid-base balance, sodium-potassium ratio, and fiber content.

Base-yielding fruits and vegetables, rich in vitamins, potassium and fiber, are staple foods of hunter-gatherer diets.

Unrefined wild plant foods like those available to contemporary hunter-gatherers typically exhibit low glycemic indices. Moreover, their diets are devoid of dairy products, such as milk, yogurt, and cottage cheese, which have low glycemic indices, but are highly insulinotropic, with an insulin index similar to that of white bread.

very important

28 According to most anthropologists and archeologists (as well as disease specialists), all of our severe diseases came from animal domestication. As the historian William H. McNeill argues in his book *Plagues and Peoples*, animal domestication created the ideal circumstances under which infectious disease could be communicated from animal herds to human populations upon a scale that, for reasons of socio-ecological dynamics, had never before been possible. McNeill in fact contends that most of the distinctive epidemic diseases of humanity, such as tuberculosis, smallpox and measles, most likely transferred to humans from animal herds. Certainly, human diseases often share a common ancestry with animal ones: measles, rinderpest and distemper, for example, are all closely related pseudo-myxoviruses.

These dietary characteristics may lower the risk of diabetes, obesity and other related syndrome X diseases by placing less stress on the pancreas to produce insulin, and preventing insulin insensitivity.

Hunter-gatherer diets generally maintain relatively high levels of monounsaturated and polyunsaturated fats, moderately low levels of saturated fats (10–15% of total food energy) as well as a low omega-6:omega-3 fatty acid ratio. Moreover, they are devoid of artificial trans fat. These nutritional factors may serve to inhibit the development of cardiovascular disease.

Fiber-rich and low-glycemic load root vegetables, such as beets, rutabagas, carrots, celeriac and turnips, are staples of the Paleolithic diet.

Dietary protein is characteristically elevated (19–35% of energy) at the expense of carbohydrate (22–40% of energy). High protein diets may have a cardiovascular protective effect and may represent an effective weight loss strategy for the overweight or obese. Furthermore, carbohydrate restriction may help prevent obesity and type II diabetes, as well as atherosclerosis.

Fruits, vegetables, lean meats, and seafood, which are staples of the hunter-gatherer diet, are more nutrient-dense than refined sugars, grains, vegetable oils, and dairy products. Consequently, the vitamin and mineral content of the diet is very high compared with a standard diet, in many cases a multiple of the RDA. Fish and seafood represent a particularly rich source of omega-3 fatty acids and other micronutrients, such as iodine, iron, zinc, copper, and selenium, which are crucial for proper brain function and development. Terrestrial animal foods, such as muscle, brain, bone marrow, thyroid gland, and other organs, also represent a primary source of these nutrients.

Because of the absence of cereals and energy-dense, nutrient-poor foods, foods which displace base-yielding fruits and vegetables, the diet produces a net base load on the body, as opposed to a net acid load. Net acid producing diets may contribute to the development of osteoporosis and renal stones, loss of muscle mass, and age-related renal insufficiency.

Fish and seafood, such as salmon, are rich sources of essential micronutrients.

Furthermore, cereal grains, legumes, and milk contain bioactive substances, such as gluten and casein, which have been implicated in the development of various health problems. Consumption of gluten, a component of certain grains, such as wheat, rye and barley, is known to have adverse health effects in individuals suffering from a range of gluten sensitivities, including coeliac disease. Since the Paleolithic diet is devoid of cereal grains, it is free of gluten. The paleodiet is also casein-free. Casein is a protein found in milk and dairy products, which may impair glucose tolerance in humans.

Compared to Paleolithic food groups, cereal grains and legumes contain relatively high amounts of antinutrients, including alkylresorcinols, alpha-amylase inhibitors, protease inhibitors, lectins and phytates, substances known to interfere with the body's absorption of many key nutrients. Molecular-mimicking proteins, which are basically made up of strings of amino acids which closely resemble those of another totally different protein, are also found in grains and legumes, as well as milk and dairy products.

It can be said then, that "civilization" has brought us closer to all types of diseases and early deaths based on what we eat. Let us look at how to take what I believe to be the best of what our science of today (in earlier Chapters on hormones, and aging) has to offer and combine it with what appears to be the proper evolutionary standard.

CHAPTER VIII

LEARNING WHAT CONSTITUTES "REAL" FOOD

You have now been exposed to a lot of scientific facts, other expert points of view, evolutionary historical knowledge, facts, and medical review, and also some rather paradoxical theories by both modern nutritionists and the Food and Drug Administration's Food Pyramid. These paradoxes seem to be squashed by the weight of the truths which we behold here within this book—truths about "diet" and what our bodies were designed to consume and what many choose to consume now in our fast-paced, commercialistic, "Techno sapiens" social experiment. These paradoxes are clearly just that—paradoxes which, once researched and reflected upon, change into the one "Human Diet," about which we have been talking. As you have seen, these "experiments" started some 10,000 years ago with the advent of plant and animal domestication and continue to this day.

Where do you begin to understand all of this in the face of grocery stores which are lined with foods which even the FDA considers unhealthy? Actually, it is quite simple. First, you want to take a look at the list below in order to get an idea of what your choices are going to look like.

The following is what I believe to be the healthiest group of proteins, carbohydrates, and fats to eat in our modern world, assuming that all animals are pastured, "free-range," not given any drugs, and are not fed any grains. My dog eats grain-free dog food, and he does his duty three times a day. I do the same, and so should you! Having one bowel movement a day or every two days is absolutely a bad idea. Grains, despite what some would have you believe, do not provide the best sources of roughage. (The order of Proteins, vegetables, and fats are random and do not mean one is better than another—that is written elsewhere in this book many places.)

BEST PROTEINS
wild fish
skinless chicken
egg whites, hard-boiled
skinless turkey
white fish
soy beans
lean beef
lean pork
tuna
yogurt

BEST VEGETABLES
all greens
peppers
asparagus
tomatoes
all squashes
yams
sweet potatoes
potatoes

ONLY STARCHES
organic brown rice

BEST FATS
raw almonds — *Not the Best.*
raw hazelnuts
avocados
pine nuts
olives
Walnuts Best
Macodamia Nuts

BEST OILS
~~canola~~
olive oil in can[29]

FRUITS

apples	blueberries	pineapple	grapes
strawberries	blackberries	watermelon	others
pears	honeydew melon	cantaloupe	

This list gives you an insight into what has stood the test of time as far as we know. Not all of these foods were around 12,000 to 40,000 years ago, of that we can be certain; however, none of these foods would summon the level of pancreatic response which is necessary for cellular uptake of pasta, bread, or other grain-based and flour-based products. The most important change in human nutrition history was the spread of the use of grains and the flour made from them. Everyone I know who eats pasta and other grain-based and flour-based foods are "addicted" to these foods. When I say addiction, I am not referring to the standard answer which I get: "I like pasta." By saying this alone, they are not simply meaning that they like pasta and make an informed choice to eat it. No, what I am saying is the same thing which people who smoke cigarettes know—their bodies needs it because of the physiological changes and addictive behavior both cigarettes and grain-based foods create. The only reason anyone smokes cigarettes or eats pasta is not because they "like it"—it is because they are addicted to the products, and their physiology is craving a fix. Their body craves them both, as does any addict. If that doesn't say addiction loud enough, then think of the processing of foods and drugs as such. In South America, the ancient aboriginals used to put the living coca leaf under their tongues for running long distances. They knew that they would get a small boost of energy from this leaf. Now, what people who make cocaine do, is to break that leaf down and make it into a paste (obviously with many leaves). They add some hydrochloric acid and some

---

29   Any time an oil which you are going to use for cooking has been exposed to UV light (the sun), that oil has begun a process of molecular change and destruction. Any type of oil which you use for cooking (only two are shown, though some people believe coconut oil is a good oil with which to cook) should come in a can or a very dark bottle.

other ethyl-type products, dry it, and put it into a microwave (or a version of this powerful radioactive wave emitter). Then they have a "brick," which is broken down into powder at some point at the street-level sale and that is how it is ingested—often in any orifice of the body. I say this because women have recently found that vaginal implanting of cocaine powder is very powerful—(this is a very stupid thing to do). So, whatever way it goes into the body, it is no longer a mere leaf that can boost your heart rate and the like, but you have a very powerful drug known as cocaine which your body gets addicted to quite easily. It is this refinement process which is the key to any addiction. You are making something in nature hundreds of times more powerful by this refining process. This is the same thing which goes on when wheat is broken down and gluten comes out as a result. Gluten is something which is so damaging to the intestinal track that anyone who eats enough of it will probably get some type of chronic illness—sometimes so bad that they can stop eating flour and still take years to get better.

Now, let's take pasta for instance. First, as explained earlier, pasta and other grain-based foods are made from the mutant grains of wheat. As stated earlier in the text, the first domesticated grains of wheat had to be taken from plants which were useless to the procreation of wheat as a living organism. Why does this matter? Think about it this way. If we, as humans, procreated mutant beings with other mutants, how long would we survive as a species? Seven generations at best.

That is not the worst of it, though. Wheat was never intended to be grown in "amber waves of grain." Mutant wheat is in those fields. On top of that, we never even eat the "whole" wheat seed anyway. We end up with the flour made from the seeds. This flour is similar to cocaine in that it has been processed. Since our pancreas was designed to send out certain amounts of insulin for wild grains, it certainly cannot be expected to send out the proper amounts for processed grains. The flour (whether it is called "whole wheat" or not) is the cocaine of the grain world, and you are addicted. Granted, the effects of cocaine are immediate and more debilitating because of the excessive amount of ethyl-type liquids used to make it. However, flour is just as bad in the long run, and here is why: the insulin is much more likely to store the flour as fat than glucose (and/or glycogen). The amount of insulin alone sends another set of cues to the hypothalamus and adrenal glands for back-up cortisol—the sledgehammer of getting refined food into fat cells and lowering dangerous blood glucose levels.

In addition, as if it mattered much a this point, there are no grains on the market which are "whole." You cannot make "whole wheat" seeds stick together, and if you could, it would be a gooey, strange-tasting mess. Thus, since you cannot eat whole wheat, what you are eating is flour. Sure, it has been dyed to look brown, and you may see some cut wheat seeds here and there in a slice of bread, but trust me—there is no such thing as "whole wheat" bread.

Since what you are eating when taking in pasta, bread, ravioli, bagels, and so forth, is actually flour, you are making your cells addicted to this refined flour—not all that dissimilar to those cells which crave cocaine once they have been exposed. Many people who start eating as I reveal in this book often go back to eat wheat, flour, or sugar, and find they have terribly bloated stomachaches along with headaches, burned tongue, and other not surprising responses. We were not designed to eat these products, so if you can get away from them for three months and then go back, your body will act adversely to them. However, most Americans (if not all) start eating these cheaply made forms of food (which I have called "faux-food" in the past) at a very young age. When you are young, you can eat all kinds of sugar, processed food, and processed grains and have little to no side effects—no overt effects other than a patch of flaky skin here and there. That is because our cells are very penetrable and easily allow nutrients in—especially when we are young. When we get older, however, our cells get harder and harder with each heavy shot of insulin the pancreas discharges into the bloodstream to store refined food as fat. Insulin is primarily a storage hormone. It stores micronutrients and macronutrients in cells and fat when we eat in excess at any one sitting and/or when grain-flour and saturated fats are eaten.

Eating flour and other grain products has more dilemmas. For one, it causes too much insulin to be secreted. Flour is just like sugar to the pancreas. It spills out too much insulin with any type of flour, even if it is "whole wheat" or "whole grain," and the insulin spikes; the flour soon is sent to fat cells, the cortisol is released to hammer down roller-coaster blood-glucose levels, and finally your intestines are left to deal with breaking down gluten, which is the sticky, gooey part of flour. That is a big culprit in many gastrointestinal issues, such as IBS (irritable bowel syndrome), acid reflux disease, and too many others to list.

Secondly, there is some form of inflammation that goes on in the body when most people eat grain-flour products. This is either because our bodies stopped organically evolving long before grains were domesticated and/or the simple fact that from the time that any American (almost any human) reaches the ripe old age of twenty, his or her body has been bombarded with so many foods made with grains and grain-flours that our immune response is that of allergic (first), then autoimmune-type response later in life. Is there a small percentage of the population who eats grains and is not affected? Probably so, but do you really want to take that chance?

If we take all foods made from grains out of our diet, then we are left with vegetables, fruits, berries, nuts, and lean animal protein sources. That may sound boring to you. However, in the upcoming pages there will be a couple of weeks of meal plans which you can follow, and I guarantee that you will lose fat, gain muscle, feel a lot more energy—and never crave grains again. That is the failure of calorie-counting, eat-anything-you-want diets! You are still a grain-flour addict!! Is there really anyone who cannot live without grains? There is two times the roughage in vegetables and fruits than is present in grains.

CHAPTER IX

UNDERSTANDING WHAT TO BUY

WHERE TO SHOP AND WHAT TO BUY

1. Shop at grocery stores which are fundamentally "organic." Although the word organic literally means "from the soil," in our post-modern era it means that more than likely the vegetables have been grown without pesticides and that the meats are non-antibiotic, non-steroidal, raised without growth hormones, and slaughtered or killed in relatively clean environments. Up here in the Northeast, we have a chain of stores called "Whole Foods." That is a very good name for a grocery store because all you want to eat are foods which have not been processed. Whole, raw, and real.

2. If you decide to eat dairy, read the following: meat, eggs, and dairy products from ***pastured*** animals are ideal for your health (according to some smarter dairy farmers). Compared with commercial products, they offer you more "good" fats and fewer "bad" fats. They are richer in antioxidants, including vitamins E, beta-carotene, and vitamin C. Furthermore, they do not contain traces of added hormones, antibiotics, or other drugs.

Below is a summary of these important benefits. Following the summary is a list of news bulletins which provide additional reasons for finding a local provider of grass-fed food.

In the 1930s, scientists and food producers were creating the first plans to take poultry off family farms and raise them in confinement. To enact their plans, they needed to create "feed rations" which would keep the birds alive and productive even though they were denied their natural diet of greens, seeds, and insects. It was a time of trial and error.

In a 1993 experiment conducted by the U.S. Department of Agriculture, breeding hens were taken off pasture and fed a wide variety of feed ingredients. When the birds were fed a diet which was exclusively soy, corn, wheat, or cottonseed meal, the chickens didn't lay eggs, or the chicks which developed from the eggs had a high rate of mortality and disease.

However, when birds were fed these same inadequate diets and put back on pasture, their eggs were perfectly normal. The pasture grasses and the bugs made up for whatever was missing in each of the highly restrictive diets.[30]

3.   Find a conscientious butcher. I have noticed that small butcher shops here and there may specialize in "pastured," non-antibiotic, non-steroidal, chicken, beef, turkey, lamb, and so on, which were not raised with growth hormones. I prefer ground pure white chicken; I make tasty, herb-laden patties from it. It turns out that this is often the purest meat out there. Don't trust meats which are in fancy packages and look perfect—they are probably filled with growth hormone and a new twist. Some large chicken companies are injecting wheat, gluten, and other sticky and thickening substances into their poultry (usually the ground chicken).

4.   If you still do not believe that grain-based foods are unhealthy, take a look at the following data which shows how grain-fed animals which you might be eating do with grains as opposed to "wild" grass and insects (their natural food).

IMPORTANT HEALTH BENEFITS OF GRASS-FED MEATS, EGGS, AND DAIRY

Lower in Fat and Calories. There are a number of nutritional differences between the meat of pasture-raised and feedlot-raised animals. To begin with, meat from grass-fed cattle, sheep, and bison is lower in total fat. If the meat is very lean, it can have one-third as much fat as a similar cut from a grain-fed animal. In fact, as you can see by the graph below, grass-fed beef can have the same amount of fat as skinless chicken breast, wild deer, or elk. Research shows that lean beef actually lowers your "bad" LDL cholesterol levels.

---

30   "The Effect of Diet on Egg Composition." *Journal of Nutrition* 6(3): 225-242. 1933.

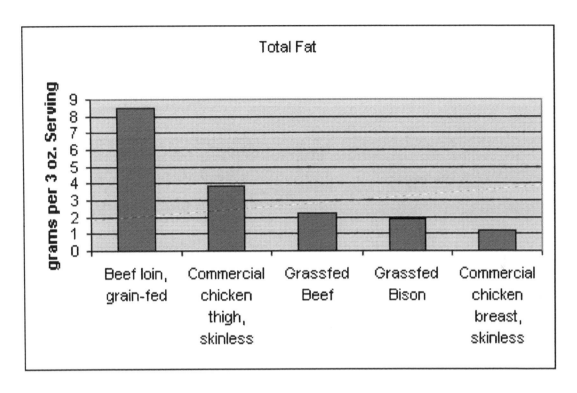

Data from J. Animal Sci 80(5):1202–11.

Because meat from grass-fed animals is lower in fat than meat from grain-fed animals, it is also lower in calories. (Fat has 9 calories per gram, compared with only 4 calories for protein and 7 grams for carbohydrates. The greater the fat content, the greater the number of calories). As an example, a 6-ounce steak from a grass-fed steer can have 100 fewer calories than a 6-ounce steak from a grain-fed steer. If you eat a typical amount of beef (66.5 pounds a year), switching to lean, grass-fed beef will save you 17,733 calories a year—without requiring any willpower or change in your eating habits. If everything else in your diet remains constant, you'll lose about six pounds a year. If all Americans switched to grass-fed meat, our national epidemic of obesity might diminish.

In the past few years, producers of grass-fed beef have been looking for ways to increase the amount of marbling in the meat in order that consumers will have a more familiar product. However, even these fatter cuts of grass-fed beef are lower in fat and calories than beef from grain-fed cattle.

Extra Omega-3s. Meat from grass-fed animals has two to four times more omega-3 fatty acids than meat from grain-fed animals. Omega-3s are called "good fats" because they play a vital role in every cell and system in your body. For example, of all the fats, they are the most heart-friendly. People who have ample amounts of omega-3s in their diet are less likely to have high blood pressure or an irregular heartbeat. Remarkably, they are 50 percent less likely to suffer a heart attack. Omega-3s are essential for your brain as well. People with a diet rich in omega-3s are less likely to suffer from depression, schizophrenia, attention deficit disorder (hyperactivity), or Alzheimer's disease.

Another benefit of omega-3s is that they may reduce your risk of cancer. In animal studies, these essential fats have slowed the growth of a wide array of cancers and also kept them from spreading. Although the human research is in its infancy, researchers have shown that omega-3s can slow or even reverse the extreme weight loss which accompanies advanced cancer and also hasten recovery from surgery.

Omega-3s are most abundant in seafood and certain nuts and seeds such as flaxseeds and walnuts, but they are also found in animals raised on pasture. The reason is simple. Omega-3s are formed in the chloroplasts of green leaves and algae. Of the fatty acids in grass, 60 percent are omega-3s. When cattle are taken off grass which is rich in omega-3s and shipped to a feedlot to be fattened on grain which is low in omega-3s, they begin losing their store of this beneficial fat. Each day that an animal spends in the feedlot, its supply of omega-3s is diminished. The graph below illustrates this steady decline.

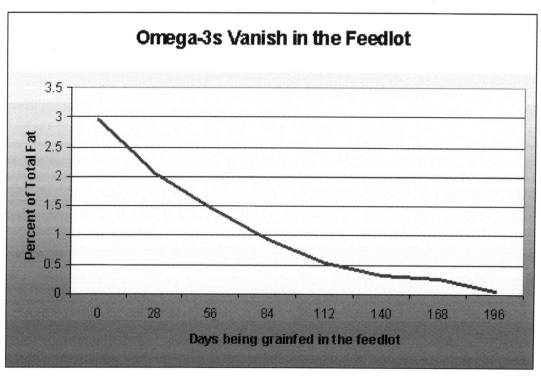

Data from J Animal Sci (1993) 71(8):2079–88.

When chickens are housed indoors and deprived of greens, their meat and eggs also become artificially low in omega-3s. Eggs from pastured hens can contain as much as ten times more omega-3s than eggs from factory hens.

It has been estimated that only 40 percent of Americans consume an adequate supply of omega-3 fatty acids, and 20 percent have blood levels so low that they cannot be detected. Switching to the meat, milk, and dairy products of grass-fed animals is one way to restore this vital nutrient to your diet.

The CLA Bonus. Meat and dairy products from grass-fed ruminants are the richest known source of another type of good fat called "conjugated linoleic acid," or CLA.

CLA is a newly discovered good fat called "conjugated linoleic acid" which may be a potent cancer fighter. In animal studies, very small amounts of CLA have blocked all three stages of cancer: 1) initiation, 2) promotion, and 3) metastasis. Most anti-cancer agents block only one of these stages. What's more, CLA has slowed the growth of an unusually wide variety of tumors, including cancers of the skin, breast, prostate, and colon.

Where do you get CLA? Many people take a synthetic version which is widely promoted as a diet aid and muscle builder. New research shows that the type of CLA in the pills may have some potentially serious side effects, including *promoting* insulin resistance, raising glucose levels, and reducing HDL (good) cholesterol.

Few people realize that CLA is also found in nature, and this natural form does not have any known negative side effects. The most abundant source of natural CLA is the meat and dairy products of grass-fed animals. Research conducted since 1999 shows that grazing animals have from three to five times more CLA than animals fattened on grain in a feedlot. Simply switching from grain-fed to grass-fed products can greatly increase your intake of CLA.

At the molecular level, CLA resembles another type of fat called "linoleic acid," or LA. (Both CLA and LA have eighteen carbon atoms and two double bonds holding the chain together. The main difference is in the placement of those bonds.) However, CLA and LA appear to have opposite effects on the human body. For example, LA promotes tumor growth, but CLA blocks it.

There are twenty-eight possible types (isomers) of CLA, each one with a slightly different arrangement of chemical bonds. The type most commonly found in meat and dairy products has double bonds between the ninth and eleventh carbon atoms and is referred to as "cis-9, trans-11 CLA" or "rumenic acid."

When ruminants are raised on fresh pasture alone, their products contain from three to five times more CLA than products from animals fed conventional diets. (A steak from the most marbled, grass-fed animals will have the most CLA because much of the CLA is stored in fat cells).

CLA may be one of our most potent defenses against cancer. In laboratory animals, a very small percentage of CLA—a mere 0.1 percent of total calories—greatly reduced tumor growth. There is new evidence that CLA may also reduce cancer risk in humans. In a Finnish study, women who had the highest levels of CLA in their diets had a 60 percent lower risk of breast cancer than those with the lowest levels. Switching from grain-fed to grass-fed meat and dairy products places women in this lowest risk category. Researcher Tilak Dhiman from Utah State University estimates that you may be able to lower your risk of cancer simply by eating the following grass-fed products each day: one glass of whole milk, one ounce of cheese, and one serving of meat. You would have to eat five times that amount of grain-fed meat and dairy products to get the same level of protection.

Vitamin E. In addition to being higher in omega-3s and CLA, meat from grass-fed animals is also higher in vitamin E. The graph below shows vitamin E levels in meat from: 1) feedlot cattle, 2) feedlot cattle which have been given high doses of synthetic vitamin E (1,000 IU per day), and 3) cattle which have been raised on fresh pasture with no added supplements. The meat from the pastured cattle is four times higher in vitamin E than the meat from the feedlot cattle and, interestingly, almost twice as high as the meat from the feedlot cattle given vitamin E supplements. In humans, vitamin E is linked with a lower risk of heart disease and cancer. This potent antioxidant may also have anti-aging properties. Most Americans are deficient in vitamin E.

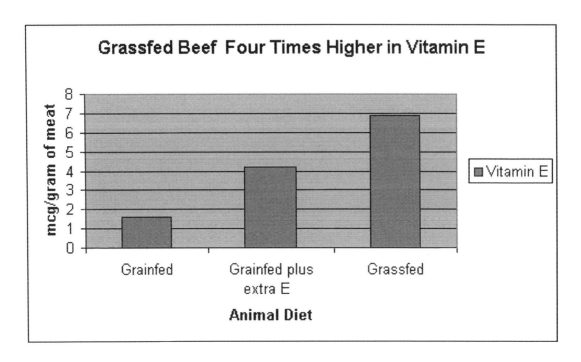

Grassfed Beef Four Times Higher in Vitamin E

Data from G. C. Smith, "Dietary Supplementation of Vitamin E to Cattle to Improve Shelf Life and Case Life of Beef for Domestic and International Markets," Colorado State University, Fort Collins, Colorado.

Free Range Eggs Are Nutritionally Superior. As it turns out, all those choices of eggs at your supermarket aren't providing you much of a choice at all.

Recent tests conducted by *Mother Earth News* magazine have shown once again that eggs from chickens which range freely on pasture provide clear nutritional benefits over eggs from confinement operations.

Mother Earth News collected samples from fourteen pastured flocks across the country and had them tested at an accredited laboratory. The results were compared to official U.S. Department of Agriculture data for commercial eggs. Results showed the pastured eggs contained an amazing:

* 1/3 less cholesterol than commercial eggs
* 1/4 less saturated fat
* 2/3 more vitamin A

- 2 times more omega-3 fatty acids
- 7 times more beta-carotene

Full results of the tests are available in the October/November 2007 issue of *Mother Earth News* or on their Web site. [31]

Lambs Raised on Pasture Are Higher in Protein, Lower in Fat. A team of scientists from the USDA compared grass-fed lambs with lambs fed grain in a feedlot. They found that "*lambs grazing pasture had 14 percent less fat and about 8 percent more protein compared to grain-fed lamb.*" The researchers acknowledged that "*consumer desires for healthier meats have shifted the emphasis to leaner, trimmer carcasses,*" and that raising more sheep on pasture will "*benefit our economy by reducing reliance upon expensive grain supplements.*"

 Eggs from Free-range Hens Are Higher in Folic Acid and Vitamin B12. Now there's another good reason to purchase eggs from pastured poultry farmers: you may be getting more folic acid and vitamin B12, two very important vitamins. This information comes from a British study published in 1974. At the time, British consumers were concerned about the trend toward factory farming. Specifically, they thought factory eggs might not be as nutritious as eggs from free-ranging birds. An elaborate study confirmed their suspicions. The eggs from free-range hens contained significantly more folic acid and vitamin B12, as you can see by the graph below.

The researchers also looked for differences in the fatty acid content of the eggs, but did not find any. Now we know why. In the 1970s, little was known about the benefits of omega-3 fatty acids, so the researchers didn't even bother to look for them in the eggs.

---

31   http://www.MotherEarthNews.com/eggs. Check Eatwild's Pastured Products Directory to find free-range eggs near you.

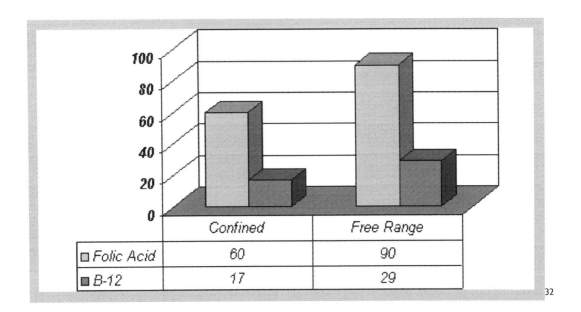

	Confined	Free Range
□ Folic Acid	60	90
■ B-12	17	29

5. Use spices such as turmeric, ginger, and rosemary, and great and healthy spicing foods such as garlic, onion, and colorful peppers. There are hundreds of other spices and herbs to help with flavoring and boost your health benefits. Read up on them and try different ones for effectiveness. Other immune boosters include:

    green tea   probiotics   cinnamon   yogurt vitamin C
    zinc   echinacea   ashwagandha

6. Find a fish market if you live on either a coastal or clean lake region. Buy only wild fish, and be sure it is as fresh as possible. Fresh fish has no odor—so that is your best indicator. If you cannot buy fresh fish, I would eat sardines packed in olive or canola oil. Oily fish are the best to eat, obviously, for the amount of DEA and DHA they contain in their fatty cells. The omega oils in oily fish will not make you fat, and they will enhance heart, arterial, and brain health.

WHICH FISH ARE SAFE TO EAT?

AVOID the following because they are overfished, or fishing is causing damaged habitats, or they are high in mercury, PCBs, or other contaminants:

---

32   A. Tolan *et al*, "Studies on the Composition of Food: The Chemical Composition of Eggs Produced under Battery, Deep Litter and Free-range Conditions," *Br. J. Nutrition*, (1974) 31:185.

- Bass, Smallmouth
- Bass, Largemouth
- Bass, Golden
- Catfish, Wild
- Caviar, Sturgeon Roe
- Caviar, Russian
- Caviar, Iranian
- Caviar, Caspian Sea
- Cod, Atlantic
- Cod, Rock
- Crab, King (imported)
- Croaker
- Dolphin-fish
- Flounder, Atlantic
- Flounder, Pacific
- Flounder, Summer or Fluke
- Flounder, Winter or Sole
- Golden Bass
- Grouper
- Haddock
- Hake, Atlantic
- Halibut, Atlantic*
- Lake Trout
- Lingcod
- Lobster, Caribbean*
- Lobster, Spiny*
- Lobster, Rock*
- Mackerel, King*
- Mackerel, Gulf*
- Mahi-Mahi
- Marlin
- Monkfish
- Orange Roughy
- Oysters, Gulf Coast*
- Patagonian Toothfish
- Pike*
- Pollock, Atlantic
- Red Snapper, Pacific*
- Rockfish
- Sablefish
- Salmon, Atlantic Wild**
- Salmon, Farmed*
- Salmon, Great Lakes**
- Sea Bass*
- Sea Bass, Chilean*
- Sea Bass, White Pacific
- Shark*
- Shrimp, Farmed
- Shrimp, Imported
- Skate
- Snapper, Golden*
- Snapper, Red*
- Snapper, Imported
- Snapper, Vermillion
- Sole, Atlantic
- Sturgeon
- Swordfish*
- Tilefish*
- Trout, Lake
- Tuna, Albacore***
- Tuna, Canned Albacore***
- Tuna, Bluefin*
- Tuna, Yellowfin*
- Walleye
- White Croaker

Quick List of ATLANTIC Fish:

- Cod, Atlantic
- Flounder, Atlantic
- Hake, Atlantic
- Halibut, Atlantic
- Pollock, Atlantic
- Salmon, Wild Atlantic**
- Sole, Atlantic

* Highest levels of mercury or PCBs!

**MOST Omega-3s per serving!

Great Lakes fish is contaminated with PCBs, DDT, and PBDE.

EAT the following because they are low in mercury, not overfished, and habitats are strong:

- Anchovies
- Arctic Char
- Bass
- Catfish, Farmed U.S.
- Char, Arctic
- Caviar, U.S.
- Caviar, French
- Caviar, Farmed
- Crawfish
- Croaker, Atlantic
- Cuttlefish, Golden

- Halibut, Wild Pacific
- Herring**
- Hoki
- Rainbow Trout
- **Salmon, Wild Pacific****
- **Salmon, Wild Alaskan****
- **Salmon, Canned****
- **Sardines****
- Striped Bass, Farmed

- Sturgeon, Farmed
- Trout, Rainbow (farmed)

Shellfish in moderation:
- Abalone, Farmed
- Clams, Farmed
- Lobster, Rock - Australian
- Lobster, Spiny - U.S.
- Shrimp, Trap Caught

**MOST Omega-3s per serving!

Unlike farmed salmon, **wild** *Alaskan salmon species* grow free of antibiotics, pesticides, synthetic coloring agents, growth hormones, and GMOs. Wild salmon is also much higher in heart and brain healthy omega-3s over farmed salmon. Moreover, the taste of wild Pacific or wild Alaskan salmon is totally delicious! It is unlike any farmed or Atlantic fish. There is a noticeable difference in flavor.

Since shellfish are bottom feeders, they should always be eaten in moderation.

Vital Choice salmon has been tested for mercury levels. Tuna and salmon are two of the best sources of omega-3s. I feel comfortable eating these fish from Vital Choice (the tuna in moderation, but the salmon regularly) because of the test results I've seen; I encourage you to research it and make your own decision about the amount you feel safe eating (wild Pacific salmon, Vital Choice wild troll-caught tuna, and wild Pacific halibut).

EAT the following cautiously and in moderation. Eat one of these only once a month, if at all, because mercury levels are moderate or the fish is coming back, but not quite fully there yet. (Please note that pregnant and nursing women should **AVOID** these fish too).

- Bass, Saltwater
- Bluefish
- Cod, Black
- Cod, Pacific
- Dover Sole
- Flounder, Pacific
- Jacksmelt
- Mackerel, Spanish**
- Mackerel, Atlantic**
- Sablefish
- Sanddabs
- Sole, Dover
- Sole, Pacific
- Tilapia, Farmed
- Tuna, Canned Light
- Tuna, Albacore.

Shellfish in moderation:
- Calamari
- Clams, Caught
- Crab, Blue
- Crab, Dungeness
- Crab, Gulf Coast
- Crab, Snow
- Lobster, American
- Lobster, Maine
- Mussels
- Oysters, Eastern
- Scallops
- Squid

7. As far as supplements go, I use pure whey (without flavoring), a multivitamin/mineral packet, and occasionally creatine. I am not one who believes that you need a lot of supplements if you are eating lots of fresh, colorful vegetables, clean meats and fish, and some spices and herbs listed on page 81. Good, fresh nuts such as pecans, almonds, and macadamia nuts are all insulin neutral, and all are good for your health in many ways.

8. Don't get caught up in dieting fads. After reading the evolutionary history of our organs, and plant and animal domestication, those facts should be enough to convince you. However, just in case you are hesitant, merely stay away from any food made or altered by man for a month. Your addictive cravings will subside, and you will find yourself eating healthier without trying. You also will be full after each meal and thus will not crave anything processed.

9. Stick to the program which you devise based on history, modern-day science, and journalistic recordings and papers.

CHAPTER X

MEAL PLANNING

BUILDING AND TRACKING LEAN MUSCLE MASS

The amount of protein which you take in with each meal will depend on your lean body mass (LBM) index and what level of athlete you are (or aspire to be). LBM is the number which is given when your body fat percentage is analyzed and deducted from your overall weight. There are many ways to calculate your body fat percentage. Obviously, one of the most accurate, but least available, is the hydrostatic tank test. Just as the name indicates, you are weighed outside of water, and then you are submerged on a scale which will give your true lean body weight. The next two or three which are credible and amazingly accurate are the infrared method and the bioelectrical impedance analysis (BIA) method, which has gained a greater reputation than it once had. These portable analysis machines have become as accurate as (and some say more accurate than) tank testing.[33] As you can read in the footnote below, there are many studies being done with BIA, and with increasingly good results. Having said that, I have owned an infrared body fat analyzer (made by Futrex[34]), and it was surprisingly accurate, although it was originally designed for measuring fat/lean mass in cattle.

---

33   K. R. Segal, M. Van Loan, P. I. Fitzgerald, J. A. Hodgdon, and T. B. Van Itallie, Division of Pediatric Cardiology, Mount Sinai School of Medicine. This study validated further the BIA method for body composition estimation. At four laboratories, densitometrically-determined lean body mass (LBMd) was compared with BIA in 1567 adults (1069 men, 498 women) aged seventeen to sixty-two years and with 3–56 percent body fat. Equations for predicting LBMd from resistance measured by BIA, height, weight, and age were obtained for the men and women. Application of each equation to the data from the other labs yielded small reductions in R values and small increases in SEEs. Some regression coefficients differed among labs, but these differences were eliminated after adjustment for differences among labs in the subjects' body fatness. All data were pooled to derive fatness-specific equations for predicting LBMd: the resulting R values ranged from 0.907 to 0.952 with SEEs of 1.97–3.03 kg. These results confirm the validity of BIA and indicate that the precision of predicting LBM from impedance can be enhanced by sex- and fatness-specific equations.

34   Futrex is the name of a company which makes infrared body fat percentage/lean muscle mass analyzers. This company's Web site is: http://www.healthfitnet.com/Products_BodyComp.htm.

The final way to find out your body fat percentage is to use skin calipers. Although very competent people in the health and fitness field seem to be able to come quite close to each other when testing for lean mass and body fat, skin calipers can be deceiving. For instance, one has to know exactly where to pinch the skin (and fat, lying atop the muscle) for both men and women— they are in two different areas, which the final of four areas needs to be examined. Unless you have no other way of testing for your lean mass, then I would make this your final recourse.

What all of this means to you is that you should establish a lean body mass index for two reasons:

1. It will tell you how much protein you should take in each day.
2. It will establish a body fat percentage number which you can use as your barometer by which to gauge progress. You must not use the scale!!! Did I say that? Yes, I did. DO NOT USE YOUR SCALE AS A BAROMETER. Use the body fat percentage and lean body mass as your means of assessing progress. Why?

First, muscle is heavier than fat. We know that for certain. Put a couple of drops of olive oil into a pot of water and watch how quickly the oil (fat) floats to the top. This is a clear indication that oil is very light in comparison to water. Over 75 percent of your body is made up of water, so please do not look at the scale for direction; use the mirror and a body fat tester.

(Look to page 39 under "Meal Balancing" for your lean body mass protein, carbohydrate and fat figures.)

When going out to eat (which I really do not recommend), the best way to think of these portions is the following:

1. Protein from lean chicken (skinless) or oily fish about the size and thickness of the palm of your hand.
2. Carbohydrates in the forms of vegetables and fruits.
    a. Vegetables should be steamed and the size of your hand spread open— about the size of a normal dining plate.
    b. One piece or one bowl of fresh fruit for dessert.
3. Fats. Be sure to tell the server that you want no added fats at all. So your chicken, fish, and occasional filet should all be cooked without any oils or fats. You can put one teaspoon of olive oil on your salad, and that is plenty per meal.

MEAL PLANNING AND COOKING

The following are a few ideas for the way to arrange your meals. Keep in mind that your portions are figured out by the last chapter, whereas these are cooking and meal planning samples. Remember two things: (1) When going out to eat, choose a piece of lean protein the size and width of the palm of your hand. Choose vegetables the size of your entire hand spread out—about a plate full of steamed green and colorful vegetables (no grains, grain products, or rice). Moreover, keep all fats to a minimum. Fat from fish is fine—fat from anything else in a restaurant is not. (2) In addition, keep in mind that you should bring at least one meal and one large snack to work with you. I have heard every excuse in the world for not doing this, and yet it is so simple to fix yourself a meal the night before and put it into a plastic container and eat that for your lunch—it is absurd to not stick with the plan because you refuse to do this.

EXAMPLES OF A FEW COMPLETE DAILY MEAL PLANS

1. <u>Day One</u>.

<u>Breakfast 6:00–7:00 a.m.</u>: Depending on your protein intake, eat anywhere from three to ten egg whites, either hard-boiled (and pop out the yolks)[35] or made in an omelet with vegetables and one teaspoon of olive or canola oil to prevent sticking to pan. Remember—just the whites! Included in this breakfast should be one to three pieces of fruit, depending on your protein/carb gram count.

<u>Snack 10:00 a.m.</u>: Once again, depending on your protein intake for the day, utilize this time accordingly. Non-fat, sugar-free yogurt is a good snack. Some almonds, pecans, or macadamia nuts with grapes is a good snack—perfectly proportioned. You could have a protein drink (whey preferred) with water and a whole apple after the drink. IMPORTANT: Do not juice your fruits and vegetables.

<u>Lunch 12:30 p.m.</u>: Grilled, plain chicken breast over greens and broccoli and a piece of fruit for dessert. Alternatively, grilled salmon with steamed green vegetables, grapes, and nuts mixed in with veggies. Use hummus for taste on steamed vegetables.[36]

<u>Snack 3:30 p.m.</u>: Small fruit plate with yogurt,[37] plain water and protein with a small piece of fruit.

---

35   See the "Specialized Recipes" section of this chapter for an interesting way to make an omelet.
36   See the "Specialized Recipes" section of this chapter for how to make homemade hummus.
37   Yogurt that is fat-free and has no flavoring has a perfect combination of protein and

<u>Dinner 6:30 p.m.:</u> Grilled or poached salmon,[38] a plate of steamed green vegetables, a large piece of fruit. Alternatively, cut-up chicken breast cooked with one teaspoon of olive oil. Mix the small chunks of chicken with lemon and your favorite herb combination for chicken. (I prefer Mrs. Dash and/or rosemary/oregano/cilantro mix, and a tiny bit of a very plain olive oil-vinaigrette. You can also add a few cut green olives and a small teaspoon of mustard). Let the chunks of chicken soak in a saucer for an hour, and then cook them in a non-stick pan to allow them to cook to a golden brown without sticking. Don't be afraid to add a little salt to your food. In addition, if you find it hard to keep eating plain, steamed vegetables, mix them up with some stewed or cooked tomatoes and add some spices. Herbs and spices are usually fine to eat. They are not calories which present any type of problem.

I have noticed over the years that when people go on a "diet," they think that they have to eat very strictly. This is not the case. As you can see, you need not eat "strictly," but rather, smart and healthy. Use mustard, lemons, and herbs for flavor. Use anything that is not made of a grain, alcohol, or fat, save for a teaspoon of olive or canola oil.

2. <u>Day Two</u>.

<u>Breakfast 6:30 a.m.:</u> Four poached eggs without the yolks. This can be done in the microwave—which has its drawbacks as far as health is concerned—or it can be done with a special poacher which the egg is put in while the metal containers sit inside boiling water. These devices are worth the money if you are going to be eating a lot of eggs and you don't like eggs hard-boiled (which is the only way that you can get all of the yolk out of an egg that is cooked).

 You can also eat what is called "steel-cut" Irish oatmeal. Although I am very adamantly against eating grains, especially wheat, there are some people who can digest these "whole"[39] oats, and they like them as an alternative to eggs and fruit each morning. On the Irish oatmeal, you can put any type of fresh fruits and fresh carbohydrates. It is the only dairy product which I advocate eating (or drinking). Yogurt contains acidophilus and many "good" bacteria for your intestinal tract, as well as being a good source of protein and carbohydrates. I would eat yogurt only on occasion—not daily. I am giving you options here, but do not eat it at every snack of every day—that would not be advisable.

38   Wild salmon is a better choice until fish farms have better regulation about the amount of metal and other harmful chemicals which the fish may be ingesting.

39   There is no such thing as "whole wheat." I have never seen it, nor would anyone eat it. They put that on wrappers around bread and on other products which they call "whole wheat," but the truth is that no one has ever eaten a slice of "whole wheat bread" bought from a store in their life. It is whole wheat flour with a few seeds, but it cannot be whole wheat. That, of course, is not the reason why wheat is so bad.

nuts to flavor it up a bit. Just be sure to have a protein drink with the proper amount of protein which correlates with the carbohydrates which you are consuming with the oatmeal and fruit.

Snack 10:00 a.m.: Sometimes the best thing for a snack is some sliced turkey and a bowl of fresh fruit. There are very few places which carry "real" turkey, but the store chain "Whole Foods" does, and I am sure there are two or three others around the country that do also. By real turkey, I mean turkey which is cooked in an oven and then left out and cooled in order to be sliced and sold by the pound (or increments thereabouts) to the public. This turkey is not processed at all. It is hard to find, but it is well worth the trouble. Most other turkey bought in stores is processed and full of chemicals and shelf-life-enhancing additives which are not good for your body.

Lunch 12:00 p.m.: Grilled chicken with salad. Eat as many uncooked vegetables in the salad as you can. Do not use so-called "iceberg" lettuce (for it has few nutrients); rather, use arugula and a dark, leafy mixture as the base which should have sliced tomatoes, sliced carrots, apples, broccoli, and many other raw vegetables. Do not hold back on eating raw vegetables—they are filled with macronutrients and micronutrients.[40] You may have an apple or pear for desert.
Snack 3:30 p.m.: A de-cored pear with non-fat cottage cheese. I would recommend that you eat cottage cheese very rarely. Although similar to yogurt, it does not contain the active "good-bacteria" which makes yogurt the preferable choice of all the dairy foods. Once in a month, this type of snack is fine.

Dinner 6:30 p.m.: Cook an entire chicken by using the following instructions. Pick a large, "all-natural" chicken (no antibiotics, no growth hormone, no steroids, and no other drugs given for growth enhancement). In addition, the chicken's package should say it was "fed and raised free-range." Once you get the chicken home, take it out of the wrapper, and pull out the internal organs bag which almost all chicken farmers and preparers stick inside the chicken. In this wrapper will be the heart, liver, and other organs. If you want to eat these, cook them in boiling hot water, and then cover and eat with the chicken. Once the bag is out (and the organs are boiled or thrown away), rinse the inside and the outside of the chicken off with cool water. Cut all of the excess fat away from the chicken. Leave the rest of the skin intact. Slice a lemon and squeeze it all over the chicken— inside and outside. (I actually rub the chicken skin with the lemon halves once all of the juice has been squeezed onto and into the chicken.) Now pick your herbs

---

40　Macronutrients are the nutrients which we call protein, carbohydrates, and fats. Micronutrients are anything from vitamins A, E, C and other antioxidants to minerals (and metals) vital for health and growth such as calcium, magnesium, zinc, and a host of others.

and spices and add. (Do not use anything such as breadcrumbs, wheat- or grain-based sauces, or anything with sugar and/or products that are not "real" foods[41]).

Many people ask me if I eat a lot of red meat. Many others assume that I eat no red meat at all. The reality is that if I feel like having a pastured cow filet, I will do so. Years ago when I first went to California to continue my path as a bodybuilder, I found that there were two schools of thought about red meat amongst professional bodybuilders.[42] First, there were those who ate four to seven pounds of red meat a day. Most of these guys were big, but they were not very well defined and did not have the type of body that I wanted to build. The other school of thought on this was that lean chicken and fish were the way to go and that eating red meat was a once-a-week occurrence.

---

41   "Real" foods are only those foods which are grown from the soil or taken from a wild or domesticated animal. All breads, pastas, cereals, and other worse items such as "yellow No. 5" and other chemically altered amino acids such as saccharine are not real food. I call all of these marvelous inventions of man "faux foods."

42   The reason which I often use professional bodybuilders as a ground to find out experiential truths is because they are used to experimenting with anything and everything in order to become more heavily muscled. This is true to this day. Bodybuilders, although often laced with drugs, are usually the most knowledgeable people on earth about diet and how it relates to muscle building—and that is one form of health in which we all should be interested.

SPECIALIZED RECIPES

One of the most important things to the success of your lifelong nutrition plan is taste. Often, what people do is diet strictly for a month or so, and then they gorge themselves with all kinds of junk. I have seen this all of my life. In fact, this is usually how a neurosis will begin. Whether it is bulimia, anorexia, distorted body image, and/or any amount of neurotic behavior, there is a diet and a culture out there waiting for you to climb down into its depths and possibly take over your life.

Having condiments to put on top of vegetables is a good thing to keep in mind. Here I am going to list a specialized type of hummus for you to make and use freely upon any of the foods that you have chosen from the list.

Hummus: Take 2½ cups of dry chickpeas and put them into a bowl of cold water to soak in the refrigerator for 12 hours. You should use three times as much water as chickpeas (in this case it would be 7½ cups of water). Take the water-filled chickpeas (after soaking for 12 hours), and bring to a boil in 11 cups of water. Add 1 teaspoon of olive (or canola) oil and 1 teaspoon of sea salt. Boil for 45 minutes and strain. Cool the chickpeas, put them into a food processor, and add the following: 1 cup of sesame oil (Goyva is best); 1½ teaspoons of garlic powder; 1½ teaspoons of onion powder; ½ cup of fresh parsley (2 tablespoons if dry); 1 teaspoon of cumin; 1 teaspoon of paprika; ½ cup of lemon juice. Blend and add 2½ cups of water and sea salt to flavor.

Lentil Soup: Take 2½ cups of dry lentils and put in cold water (in refrigerator) for 12 hours. Drain water. Put (now) 5 cups of lentils into a large pot. Add 1 teaspoon of sea salt, 1 tablespoon of olive oil, and pour in 15 cups of water. Heat on medium flame for 35–45 minutes. Drain water again and place lentils in a large bowl. In the same pot, now on low heat, add the following: 3 cups of sweet onions; 3 cups of sliced tomatoes; 1 can of tomato sauce; 1 teaspoon of garlic powder; 1 teaspoon of onion powder; 1 teaspoon of sea salt; and 3 cups of water. Blend the entire mixture by hand until it is smooth. Now add lentils to the mix and cook on low flame for 45 minutes.

Great Omelet: Preheat oven to 400 degrees. Take an iron pan and put on stovetop (low heat). Add 1 cup of onions and 1 teaspoon of olive oil and let simmer a few minutes. Now add 2 cups of sliced plum tomatoes and bring heat up until water evaporates. In another pot, cook 2 whole, fresh spinach leaves. Drain water. In another large, deep iron pan, add 9 beaten egg whites (real eggs, not that synthetic stuff), add spinach, and add ½ teaspoon of sea salt. Now put the entire mixture in your deep iron pan and place into preheated oven. Cook for 20 minutes; take pan out and stir vigorously so that all the egg whites will be cooked. Now place back in the oven for ten minutes and remove.[43] ENJOY!

A key point to remember: this diet is perfect for building muscle and reducing body fat. Those who want to get as lean as possible (i.e., bodybuilders, models, actors, and so forth) should only eat protein and vegetables, with occasional fruits and nuts. It is only when eating this way that you will "see" your abdominals. Having stated this, it is not a good idea to eat this strictly all year round.

---

43   Depending on your lean mass, use eggs appropriately. There are about 7–9 grams of protein in a regular large egg.

CHAPTER XI

FINAL THOUGHTS

There is no doubt that some of you will read this book and continue eating the way that every average, uninformed American does. Some of you will continue to eat cereal for breakfast, followed by fatty, greasy sausage and cheese-filled white rolls for lunch, and pizza for your final meal of the day. A few of you may live into your eighties or even nineties and never have a problem, even with that horrible diet. If you want to roll the dice and play worse than Russian roulette odds, that is fine by me—that is the America in which we live. You are left with choices; however, we are all being led down a very unhealthy, deleterious path, by not only advertisers, but I dare say the FDA and the U.S. Department of Agriculture. It is all about money and how best to use our natural resources, and one of the biggest ones is the massive amount of wheat and other grains which farmers grow here in the U.S. I have no agenda here—I don't want to take money away from farmers. I am merely stating the facts as I see them.

Having said all of this—from our ancient ancestors and what they ate, to what anthropologists have learned, through what I have learned and written about here—it is my sincere hope that most of you will see that what you are eating could be slowly, but surely, killing you. There is no question that food and air are paradoxical necessities of life (you would die quickly without them, but you make 90 percent of all of the free radicals in your life with the utilization of them). However, the difference between someone who eats the type of diet presented here (which I have figured out to be ideal for our body's longevity, vitality, strength, stamina, and health) and the diet of post-modern "*Techno sapiens*," which amounts to a mixture of "faux foods," grain flours and grain-flour products, fried foods, and cheesy, chocolaty (delicious), but deadly foods, are like the difference between living for longevity, health, and vibrancy, and living only for the here and now, instant gratification, and more likely than not, a very short future. In the end, it is up to each of us to make our own choices and live with the consequences, which will be determined by exactly how these choices you make will control your destiny as either a healthy, vibrant, wise older person, or one dying at fifty with multiple ailments.

In this book, you have all that you could ever need to know in order to understand and explain why and how you should eat. There can be no question that plant domestication has brought wealth and food to people all over the world—and that agriculture will continue to enjoy the fruits of their labor in the future (which include both government subsidies and foreign imports). Having said that, there can't be any question about the fact that we simply stopped organically evolving long before the invention of domesticated grains, grain-based foods, and grain flours. With this knowledge, we have to begin the road leading to a better dietary foundation— that of pre-agricultural man, which has been described in this book.

Interestingly, while I was writing the early chapters of this book, a person quite quickly said after reading them: "*Are you making a case against veganism and vegetarianism?*" I did not think about it that way; however, we did evolve as carnivorous omnivores, and we should really look to the past and present to find our future. We must start raising real wild animals again—all meats, not just beef, but wild and "free-range" chickens and other animals—in order that they can be contained only by distant fences, not by a narrow confinement and a pseudo-existence. We need to go back to allowing the animals which we slaughter and eat to live a life full of energy and vibrancy before they are put in front of us to eat. We also must learn to clean up the great oceans in order that the fish which are wild can be caught and sold without mercury and other harmful metals inside of them—which we then eat. I do not know all of the answers, but I do know that we have to begin to pull back the curtain and reveal who the real "wizard" is and to find that "the devil is in the details." These would be the grains and grain-flour-based foods with which people are killing themselves—the very parts of the food pyramid of which the government tells each of us to eat the most.

In the end, we have to look at our entire food industry and look closely at how it is making our kids sick with type II diabetes and other diseases once thought of for those of fifty or greater. Our food industry is killing men and women at mid-life with horrible chronic illnesses which started decades before. In the end, our food industry is robbing all of us of the ability to live to that golden mark which so many scientists, geneticists, and sociologists talk of now: 120 years.

It is my hope that you can make some important changes in both your eating habits and the eating habits of those who may depend on you to make those choices for them. As always, my best to each and every one of you, and may you all be healthy, wealthy, and above all, be wise, for those who become wise are those who will not only have the ability to live longer, but they will be able to point the way for those who cannot see where the food industry is taking most of us.

It is also my hope that those of you who learned something from this book will actually follow this relatively easy system of nutrition and pass it along to those who are not aware of the information which is contained within these pages. Thank you for giving me the opportunity to share these thoughts and my lifelong research into the magnificent human body.

THE FUTURE

Some of you may believe that I might have the novel and romantic notion of living in some far-off land where I am safe from the grain industry, powerful lobbyists, pollutants, metals in fish, sugar, and processed "faux foods," a place where we can live like our Paleolithic ancestors. Nothing could be further from the truth. My favorite place to live is New York City. I love to be around people who have vibrancy and energy, and there are no places on earth left where one could live like our ancient ancestors, anyways. Perhaps there are a few aboriginal tribes in the Amazon Basin, Australia, New Zealand, or a remote part of Africa who still know the ways of their ancestors; however, the truth is that I want to be a "change agent" for the good of our up-and-coming generations. I do not want another generation of kids growing up eating mounds of cereal and sugar as it bashes their brains and nervous systems into near submission on the one hand, and delivers them a life of sure hyperactivity (and Ritalin and other drugs) and addiction on the other. I really do not want to take "fun" away from people. If anything, I want them to enjoy their lives to the fullest, and that is why I am in such dismay over the fact that people in our culture think that food is their number one source of "pleasure." I can understand enjoying your meals, because I know that I do—very much so. I love to eat, but I won't touch something which will set off the genetic predisposition in my nervous system which doctors call multiple sclerosis (which I have, but under control). I also want to keep my body and brain in tip-top shape, and exercise and diet are the two greatest influential factors in all of our lives which we can control.

I think that to really understand the harm which grain-based foods, processed food, and sugar has on our cells is rather easy. Believe it or not, sugar, grain-based foods, and processed foods kill cells faster than just about any vice a person can consider. Now, there are some studies which I have pointed to regarding cereals and child behavior, and I am in no way saying that you might just as well smoke crack and give up donuts, but you can rest assured that the more processed, grain-based, sugary foods you eat, the faster your cells will age (and die).

As I write this final thought, it is my hope that the total consciousness of America will demand a better way of eating. The branding tricks which so many companies play are very insidious and border on illegal. Why? Money, image, branding, greed, and deception in marketing are capitalism's worst components. Be very aware of what you purchase in the future. Try to write congressional leaders to make companies not only put ingredients on labels, but stop labeling items with shrewd and manipulative verbiage. Ask them to make it clear how the chickens, pigs, lamb, and cows were fed and raised. Make it clear as to what they drank and what type of lands they were able to roam (if any).

There are so many people buying "organic" this or that without knowing what that particular company or store means by "organic." Be aware that ground chicken produced by major companies is often laced with wheat to allow the ground chicken to stick together better when made into patties. Be aware of the difference between products that are labeled "no growth hormone or steroids" and animals which are clean of those drugs, and in addition are pastured instead of harnessed all their lives.

The future truly is in the past, and I submit to you that the sooner you get yourself onto the path of eating very cleanly, the sooner you will shed fat, gain muscle, be healthy, and have vitality.

As always, it is my sincere hope that this book has brought insight on a very difficult subject in our country.

Thank you.

All the best,

Paul T. Burke, M.Ed., PhD*

At home in Lincoln, Massachusetts

*(candidate)

NOTES

1. There are many wonderful books about American Indian myths, as there are for those indigenous cultures world wide. I highly suggest reading "The Plains Indians," by Paul Howard Carlson. At Amazon: http://www.amazon.com/s/ref=nb_ss_b_0_15?url=search-alias%3Dstripbooks&fieldkeywords=the+plains+indians&sprefix=The+Plains+Ind. I also highly recommend that you read "Black Elk Speaks, by John G. Neihardt, at Amazon: http://www.amazon.com/s/ref=nb_ss_b_1_12?url=search-alias%3Dstripbooks&field-keywords=black+elk+speaks+neihardt&sprefix=Black+Elk+Sp. This is truly a book about a shaman who had a "dream," which became a *myth*. All religions are based on earlier mythologies. Contrary to what some may believe a myth is not something that is "false," but rather something which becomes a ritual (and/or aboriginal story—passed down over millennia).

2. E.O. Wilson's works can be found on three pages of www.Amazon.com, beginning with this page: http://www.amazon.com/s/ref=nb_ss_gw?url=search-alias%3Dstripbooks&field-keywords=E.O.+Wilson Wilson's Biodiversity website is; http://saveamericasforests.org/wilson/intro.htm

3. Jared Diamond's Books can be found on www.amazon.com, beginning with this page: http://www.amazon.com/s/ref=nb_ss_gw_0_10?url=search-alias%3Dstripbooks&field-keywords=jared+diamond&sprefix=Jared+Diam. His works helped greatly in understanding how Eurasia developed from the first African Hominoids.

4. Joseph Campbell was a highly respected professor, mythologist, archeologist, and a wealth of "Old World" knowledge. You can purchase his books at www.amazon.com on page: http://www.amazon.com/s/ref=nb_ss_gw_0_6?url=search-alias%3Dstripbooks&field-keywords=joseph+campbell&sprefix=Joseph

Campbell also has a set of video/CD's which are very informative. They were filmed with Bill Moyers, just before Campbell's death. If you are interested in learning more about our ancient ancestors, read all of Campbell's books and purchase these wonderfully meaningful DVDs of his last interview, by Moyers.

5.   Although I do not agree with his "dietary plan," I do have faith in some of his anaerobic/aerobic exercise beliefs. Dr. Al Sears is a cardiologist. Read his studies and books online: http://www.alsearsmd.com/content/index. php?id=116 and on www.amazon.com page: http://www.amazon.com/s/ ref=nb_ss_gw?url=search-alias%3Dstripbooks&field-keywords=Dr.+Al+Sears &x=13&y=19

TVA another good fat in grass-fed products?

Evidence is mounting that dairy products from grass-fed cows supply yet another "good" fat to our diet—trans-vaccenic acid or TVA. Technically, TVA is classified as a "trans-fatty acid," a type of fat nutritionists tell us to avoid. However, TVA appears to behave differently from the man-made fat which comes from the hydrogenization of vegetable oil. Unlike the trans-fatty acids found in fast foods and margarine, TVA is not linked with an increased risk of cardiovascular disease and may help inhibit tumor growth and obesity.

Interestingly, TVA may perform these feats by being converted into CLA in our own bodies. In fact, dairy scientist David Schingoethe from South Dakota State University suggests that eating diary foods high in TVA may be a more effective way to increase CLA levels than ingesting CLA itself.

Schingoethe and colleagues are experimenting with increasing TVA in dairy cows by feeding them fish meal and soybeans. However, raising cows on fresh pasture and withholding all grain may prove just as effective. In fact, grass-fed cows produce milk which is naturally high in both CLA and TVA, a potentially lifesaving combination. Stay tuned!

The deadliest form of E. *Coli* is more common than originally thought. Fortunately, grass-fed animals are much less likely to transmit the disease.

A study in the March 28th, 2000 issue of the Proceedings of the *National Academy of Sciences* reports that as many as one out of every three cattle may play host to the deadliest strain of E. *coli* bacteria (0157:H). This is ten times higher than earlier estimates.

As explained in more detail in **Why Grassfed Is Best!**, feeding cattle their natural diet of grass instead of grain greatly reduces the risk of disease transmission. Why? First, it keeps the overall bacteria count low. Second, it prevents the bacteria from becoming acid resistant. Acid-resistant bacteria are far more likely to survive the acidity of our normal digestive juices and cause disease. The first graph below illustrates the absolute numbers of E. *coli* bacteria found in grass-fed versus grain-fed animals. The second graph shows how many of the bacteria are likely to withstand our gastric juices. (Note: Grass-fed animals have so few acid-resistant bacteria that the number fails to register on the scale of the graph).

One of the lead researchers on the project, USDA microbiologist James Russell, told a reporter for *Science Magazine*, "*We were absolutely shocked by the difference. WE never found an animal that didn't agree with the trend.*"

You should still take the normal precautions when handling and cooking grass-fed meat, however. As few as ten E. *coli* bacteria can cause disease in people with weakened immune systems.

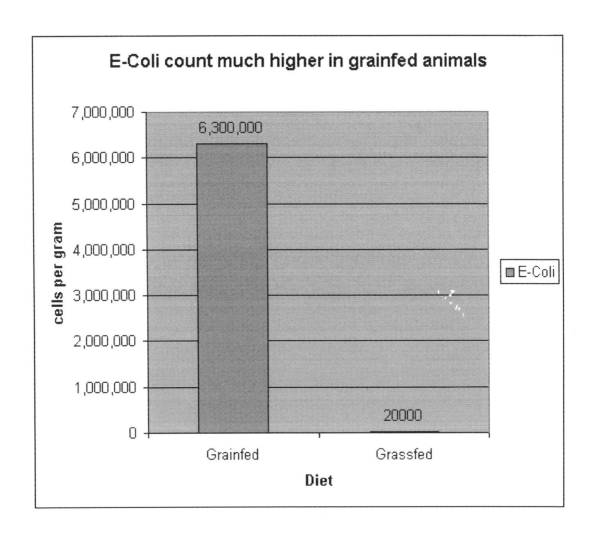

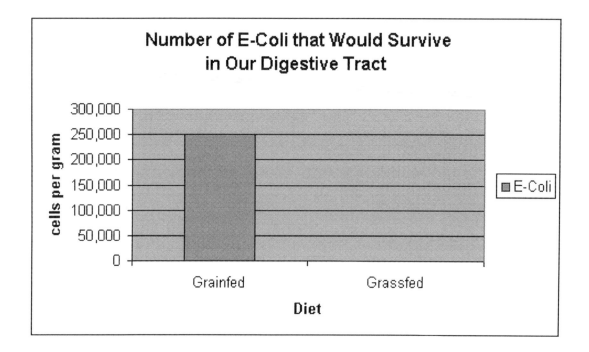

(Diez-Gonzalez, F., et al. (1998). "Grain-feeding and the dissemination of acid-resistant Escherichia coli from Cattle." Science 281, 1666-8.)

BIBLIOGRAPHY

Steckel, Richard H. (Richard Hall), 1944-
New Light on the "Dark Ages": The Remarkably Tall Stature of Northern European Men during the Medieval Era
Social Science History - Volume 28, Number 2, Summer 2004, pp. 211-228
Duke University Press

Jones, Steven, Martin, Robert and Pilbeam; *The Cambridge Encyclopedia of Human Evolution*, Cambridge University Press, 1993.

Austad, S.N. 1997. *Why We Age*. New York: John Wiley & Sons.

Baynes, J.W., and V.M. Monnier, Eds. 1989. *The Maillard Reaction in Aging, Diabetes, and Nutrition*. Alan R. Liss, New York:

Bernardis, L.L., and P.J. Davis. 1996. "Aging and the Hypothalamus." *Physical Behavior* (59: 523-536).

Burke, Paul T. "Food and Hormonal Communication." *Exercise for Men Only.*

_____. "The Markers of Aging." *Exercise For Men Only.*

_____. "Muscular Arms for the Man Over 40." *Exercise For Men Only.*

_____. "Nutritional News: Understanding Creatine." *Men's Exercise.*

_____. "The Paradox of Exercise." *Exercise For Men Only.*

_____. "Slowing Down The Aging Process." *Exercise for Men Only.*

_____. "The Synergy of Food and Exercise." *Exercise For Men Only.*

_____. "Understanding the Biological Markers of Aging." *Exercise For Men Only.*

_____. "Understanding energy In Relationship to Exercise." *Exercise For Men Only.*

_____. "Youthful Energy." *Exercise For Men Only.*

_____. "The Zone Diet, Part I." *Men's Exercise.*

_____. "The Zone Diet, Part II." *Men's Exercise.*

Butler, George, Haines. 1975. *Pumping Iron*, New York: Simon & Schuster.

Butler, George, and Gerome Gary. 2003. *Pumping Iron, The 25th Anniversary Edition*. New York: Simon & Schuster.

Butler, Tom, and George Gaines. 1974. *Pumping Iron*. New York: Simon & Schuster.

Columbo, Franco and George Fels. 1978. *Coming on Strong*, Chicago: Contemporary Books.

_____. 1979. *Winning, Body Building*, Chicago: Contemporary Books.

Columbo, Franco, D.C., with Richard Tyler, 1979. Chicago: Contemporary Books.

Crist, D. M., G.T. Peake, P.A. Eagan, and D.L. Waters. 1988. "Body composition response to exogenenous GH during training in highly conditioned adults." *Journal of Applied Physiology* 65: 579-584.

Erasmus, Udo. 1993. *Fats That Heal, Fats That Kill: The Complete Guide to Fats, Oils, Cholesterol and Human Health*. Burnaby, BC, Canada: Alive Books.

Felig, P., J.D. Baxter, and L.A. Frohman. 1995. *Endocrinology and Aging*, 3rd. Ed. New York: McGraw-Hill.

Leigh, Wendy. 1990. *Arnold: An Unauthorized Biography*. Congdon & Weed, Inc.

Little, William, H.W. Fowler, and Jessie Coulins. 1973. *The Oxford English Dictionary*. London: Oxford UP.

Murray, Michael T., N.D., 1991. *Encyclopedia of Natural Medicine*. Rocklin, CA: Prima Publishing.

_____. 1996. Encyclopedia of Nutritional Supplements. Rocklin, CA: Prima Publishing.

Parr, T. 1996. "Insulin exposure controls the rate of mammalian aging." *Mechanics of Aging and Development* (88: 75-82).

Roth, J.S., M. Gluck, R.S. Yalow, and S.A. Berson. 1964. "The influence of blood glucose on the plasma concentration of growth hormone." *Diabetes* (13: 335-361).

Schonfield, J.G. 1970. "Prostaglandin E1 and the release of growth hormone in vitro." *Nature* (228: 179).

Simon & Schuster.

Sears, Barry. 1999, *The Anti-Aging Zone*, New York: Harper Collins.

_____. 1996. *The Zone*. New York: Harper Collins.

"Superoxide Dimutase (SOD)" Medline Plus, National Library of Medicine Web site, http://www.nlm.nih.gov/medlineplus/mplusdictionary.html

Thissen, J.P., J.M. Ketelslegers, and L.E. Underwood. 1994. "Nutrition regulation of the insulin-like growth factors." *Endocrine Review* (15: 80-101).

Teihard de Chardin, *The Phenomenon of Man*, translated by Bernard Wall, forwarded by Julian Huxley, William Collins & Sons Ltd., London 1959.

W.S. Penn, editor, *The Telling of the World, Native American Stories and Art*, Stewart, Tabori & Chang, New York, 1993

Albert Einstein, *Relativity*, Crown Publishers Inc., 1961.

W.S. Penn, editor, *The Telling of the World, Native American Stories and Art*, Stewart, Tabori & Chang, New York, 1993

Steve Jones, Robert Martin, David Pilbeam. Executive Editor, Sarah Bunney, Forward by Richard Dawkins. *The Cambridge Encyclopedia of Human Evolution*, Cambridge University Press, 1992.

R.D. Martin, *Primates Origin and Evolution*, Princeton University Press, 1990.

J. Reader, *Missing Links: The Hunt for Earliest Man*, Penguin Books, London, 1998.

R. Milner, *The Encyclopedia of Evolution*, Humanity's Search for its Origins, New York, 1990.

R.E. Passingham, *The Human Primate*, Oxford and San Fransico, 1982.

I. Tattersall, *Encyclopedia of Human Evolution and Prehistory*, Garland Press, New York and London, 1988.

M.W. Stricken, *Evolution*, Jones and Bartlette, Boston, 1990.

J. Gowlette, *Ascent to Civilization*: The Archeology of Early Humans, Maidenhead and New York: McGraw Hill, 1993.

J. Diamond, *The Third Chimpanzee*, Harper Collins, New York, 1998

Jared Diamond, *Guns, Germs, and Steel*, W.W. Norton & Co., New York 1992.

Kent Flannery, "The origins of agriculture," Annual Reviews of Anthropology 2:271-310.

Jack Harlan, *Crops and Man*, 2nd. ed. (Madison, Wis. American Society of Agronomy, 1992.

Sun Bear, Waban Wind, *Dreaming with the Wheel*, Simon & Schuster, New YorK, 1994

.Thomas E. Mails, *The Mystic Warriors Of The Plains*, Mallard Press, 1972.

Natalie Curtis, *The Indians Book*, Authentic Native American Legends, Lore&Music, Bonanza Books, 1987.

Duane Champagne, Chronology Of Native North American History, Gale Research Inc., 1994.

Timothy Severen, *Vanishing Primitive Man*, American Heritage Publishing, New York, 1973

W.S. Penn, *The Telling of The World*, A Fair Street/Welcome Book, New York, 1990.

Felig, P., J.D. Baxter and L.A. Frohman. *Endocrinology and Aging*, 3rd. ed. McGraw- Hill, New York, NY (1995).

Austad, S.N. *Why We Age*. John Wiley & Sons, New York, NY (1997).

Baynes, J.W., and V.M. Monnier, eds. *The Maillard Reaction in Aging, Diabetes, and Nutrition*. Alan R. Liss, New York (1989).

Sears, B. *The Anti-Aging Zone*, Harper Collins, New York, NY (1999).

Bernardis, L.L., and P.J. Davis. "Aging and the Hypothalamus." *Physical Behavior* 59: 523-536 (1996).

Parr, T. "Insulin exposure controls the rate of mammalian aging." *Mechanics of Aging and Development* 88: 75-82 (1996).

Crist, D. M., G.T. Peake, P.A. Eagan, and D.L. Waters. "Body composition response to exogenenous GH during training in highly conditioned adults." *Journal of Applied Physiology* 65: 579-584 (1988).

Roth, J.S., M. Gluck, R.S. Yalow, and S.A. Berson. "The influence of blood glucose on the plasma concentration of growth hormone." *Diabetes* 13: 335-361 (1964).

Schonfield, J.G. "Prostaglandin E1 and the release of growth hormone in vitro." *Nature* 228: 179 (1970).

Thissen, J.P., J.M. Ketelslegers, and L.E. Underwood. "Nutrition regulation of the insulin-like growth factors." *Endocrine Review* 15: 80-101

References:

1. Kozlowska, Z: (1991). Results of investigation on children with coeliakia treated many years with glutethen free diet Psychiatria Polska. 25(2),130-134.
2. Saukkonen T, Vaisanen S, Akerblom HK, Savilahti E. Coeliac disease in children and adolescents with type 1 diabetes: a study of growth, glycaemic control, and experiences of families. Acta Paediatr. 2002;91(3):297-302.
3. Spiekerkoetter U, Seissler J, Wendel U. General Screening for Celiac Disease is Advisable in Children with Type 1 Diabetes. Horm Metab Res. 2002 Apr;34(4):192-5.
4. Barera G, Bonfanti R, Viscardi M, Bazzigaluppi E, Calori G, Meschi F, Bianchi C, Chiumello G. Occurrence of celiac disease after onset of type 1 diabetes: a 6-year prospective longitudinal study. Pediatrics. 2002 May;109(5):833-8.
5. Hansen D, Bennedbaek FN, Hansen LK, Hoier-Madsen M, Hegedu LS, Jacobsen BB, Husby S. High prevalence of coeliac disease in Danish children with type 1 diabetes mellitus. Acta Paediatr. 2001 Nov;90(11):1238-43.
6. MacFarlane AJ, Burghardt KM, Kelly J, Simell T, Simell O, Altosaar I, Scott FW. A type 1 diabetes-related protein from wheat (triticum aestivum): cDNA clone of a wheat storage globulin, Glb1, linked to islet damage. J Biol Chem. 2002 Oct 29.
7. Paul, K., Todt, J., Eysold, R. (1985) [EEG Research Findings in Children with Celiac Disease According to Dietary Variations]. Zeitschrift der Klinische Medizin. 40, 707-709.
8. Grech, P.L., Richards, J., McLaren, S., Winkelman, J.H. (2000) Psychological sequelae and quality of life in celiac disease. Journal of Pediatric Gastroenterology and Nutrition 31(3): S4
9. Reichelt, K., Ekrem, J., Scott, H. (1990b). Gluten, Milk Proteins and Autism: DIETARY INTERVENTION EFFECTS ON BEHAVIOR AND PEPTIDE SECRETION. Journal of Applied Nutrition. 42(1), 1-11.
10. Reichelt, K., Knivsberg, A., Lind, G., Nodland, M. (1991). Probable etiology and Possible Treatment of Childhood Autism. Brain Dysfunction. 4, 308-319.
11. Wahab PJ, Meijer JW, Dumitra D, Goerres MS, Mulder CJ. Coeliac disease: more than villous atrophy. Rom J Gastroenterol. 2002 Jun;11(2):121-7.
12. Catassi C, Ratsch IM, Gandolfi L, Pratesi R, Fabiani E, El Asmar R, Frijia M, Bearzi I, Vizzoni L. Why is coeliac disease endemic in the people of the Sahara? Lancet. 1999 Aug 21;354(9179):647-8.
13. Discontinuation on Cerebral Blood Flow in Prepubescent Boys with Attention Deficit Hyperactivity Disorder. J Nucl Med. 2002 Dec;43(12):1624-1629.

14. Case records of the Massachusetts General Hospital. Weekly clinicopathological exercises. Case 43-1988. A 52-year-old man with persistent watery diarrhea and aphasia. N Engl J Med. 1988 Oct 27;319(17):1139-48.

15. Hadjivassiliou M, Boscolo S, Davies-Jones GA, Grunewald RA, Not T, Sanders DS, Simpson JE, Tongiorgi E, Williamson CA, Woodroofe NM. The humoral response in the pathogenesis of gluten ataxia. Neurology. 2002 Apr 23;58(8):1221-6.

16. Hadjivassiliou M, Grunewald RA, Davies-Jones GA. Gluten sensitivity as a neurological illness. J Neurol Neurosurg Psychiatry. 2002 May; 72(5):560-3. Review.

17. Youdim MB, Yehuda S. The neurochemical basis of cognitive deficits induced by brain iron deficiency: involvement of dopamine-opiate system. Cell Mol Biol (Noisy-le-grand). 2000 May; 46(3):491-500.

18. Otero GA, Aguirre DM, Porcayo R, Fernandez T. Psychological and electroencephalographic study in school children with iron deficiency. Int J Neurosci. 1999 Aug; 99(1-4):113-21.

19. Guesry P. The role of nutrition in brain development.

20. Prev Med. 1998 Mar-Apr; 27(2):189-94. Review.

21. Holmes GK. Coeliac disease and Type 1 diabetes mellitus - the case for screening. Diabet Med. 2001 Mar; 18(3):169-77. x

22. Scott FW, Rowsell P, Wang GS, Burghardt K, Kolb H, Flohe S. Oral exposure to diabetes-promoting food or immunomodulators in neonates alters gut cytokines and diabetes. Diabetes. 2002 Jan;51(1):73-8.

23. Scott FW, Cloutier HE, Kleemann R, Woerz-Pagenstert U, Rowsell P, Modler HW, Kolb H. Potential mechanisms by which certain foods promote or inhibit the development of spontaneous diabetes in BB rats: dose, timing, early effect on islet area, and switch in infiltrate from Th1 to Th2 cells. Diabetes. 1997 Apr; 46(4):589-98.

24. Bryngelsson, Susanne; & Asp, Nils-Georg (March 2005). "Popular diets, body weight and health: What is scientifically documented?". *Scandinavian Journal of Food & Nutrition* **49** (1): 15–20. doi:10.1080/11026480510031990, http://journals.sfu.ca/coaction/index.php/fnr/article/viewFile/1515/1383.

25. Cordain, Loren (Summer 2002). "The nutritional characteristics of a contemporary diet based upon Paleolithic food groups" (PDF). *Journal of the American Nutraceutical Association* **5** (5): 15–24, http://www.ana-jana.org/Journal/journals/ACF5FB7.pdf.

26. Lindeberg S, Cordain L, Eaton SB (September 2003). "Biological and clinical potential of a Paleolithic diet" (PDF). *Journal of Nutritional and Environmental Medicine* **13** (3): 149–60. doi:10.1080/13590840310001619397, http://www.thepaleodiet.com/articles/J%20Nutr%20Environ%20Med%202003.pdf.

27. Voegtlin, Walter L. (1975). *The stone age diet: Based on in-depth studies of human ecology and the diet of man.* Vantage Press. ISBN 0533013143.

28. .Milton, Katharine (2002). "Hunter-gatherer diets: wild foods signal relief from diseases of affluence (PDF)", in Ungar, Peter S. & Teaford, Mark F.: *Human Diet: Its Origins and Evolution.* Westport, CT: Bergin and Garvey, 111–22. ISBN 0897897366.

29. Kligler, Benjamin & Lee, Roberta A. (eds.) (2004). "Paleolithic diet", *Integrative medicine.* McGraw-Hill Professional, 139–40. ISBN 007140239X.

30. Eaton SB, Cordain L, Lindeberg S (February 2002). "Evolutionary Health Promotion: A consideration of common counter-arguments" (PDF). *Preventive Medicine* **34** (2): 119–23. doi:10.1006/pmed.2001.0966. PMID 11817904, http://www.thepaleodiet.com/articles/Counter%20Arguments%20Paper.pdf.

31. Lindeberg S, Jönsson T, Granfeldt Y, Borgstrand E, Soffman J, Sjöström K, Ahrén B (September 2007). "A Palaeolithic diet improves glucose tolerance more than a Mediterranean-like diet in individuals with ischaemic heart disease" (PDF). *Diabetologia* **50** (9): 1795–807. doi:10.1007/s00125-007-0716-y. PMID 17583796, http://www.springerlink.com/content/h7628r66r0552222/fulltext.pdf.

32. Eaton, S. Boyd (February 2006). "The ancestral human diet: what was it and should it be a paradigm for contemporary nutrition?". *Proceedings of the Nutrition Society* **65** (1): 1–6. doi:10.1079/PNS2005471. PMID 16441938, http://journals.cambridge.org/action/displayFulltext?type=6&fid=814480&jid=&volumeId=&issueId=01&aid=814476&fulltextType=MR&fileId=S00296 65106000012.

33. Elton, S. (2008). "Environments, adaptations and evolutionary medicine: Should we be eating a 'stone age' diet?", in O'Higgins, P. & Elton, S.: *Medicine and Evolution: Current Applications, Future Prospects.* London: Taylor and Francis. ISBN 1420051342.

34. Milton, Katharine (March 2000). "Hunter-gatherer diets—A different perspective". *American Journal of Clinical Nutrition* **71** (3): 665–67. PMID 10702155, http://www.ajcn.org/cgi/content/full/71/3/665.

35. Ströhle A, Wolters M, Hahn A (January 2007). "Carbohydrates and the diet-atherosclerosis connection—More between earth and heaven. Comment on the article "The atherogenic potential of dietary carbohydrate"". *Preventive Medicine* **44** (1): 82–4. doi:10.1016/j.ypmed.2006.08.014. PMID 16997359.

36. Jeanie Lerche, Davis (March 15, 2002). "The Caveman Diet". MedicineNet. Retrieved on January 19, 2008.

37. Nestle, Marion (March 2000). "Paleolithic diets: a sceptical view". *Nutrition Bulletin* **25** (1): 43–7. doi:10.1046/j.1467-3010.2000.00019.x.

38. Moffat, Tina (2001). "Book Review—Evolutionary Aspects of Nutrition and Health: Diet, Exercise, Genetics and Chronic Disease". *Human Biology* **73** (2): 327–29. doi:10.1353/hub.2001.0021, http://muse.jhu.edu/journals/human_biology/v073/73.2moffat.html.

39. Jacks, Gunnar (August 22–28, 2005). "Paleolitisk kost—ett realistiskt alternativ för alla? [Alt. title: Paleolithic diet—a realistic alternative for everyone?]" (in Swedish) (PDF). *Läkartidningen* **102** (34): 2334. PMID 16167639, http://www.lakartidningen.se/store/articlepdf/1/1852/LKT0534s2334_2334.pdf.
40. Fallon, Sally; Enig, Mary G. (January 1, 2000). "Caveman Cuisine". Weston A. Price Foundation. Retrieved on January 19, 2008.
41. "Functional and Structural Comparison of Man's Digestive Tract with that of a Dog and Sheep". Retrieved on January 19, 2008.
42. Audette, Ray V.; Gilchrist, Troy; Audette, Raymond V.; & Eades, Michael R. (2000). *Neanderthin : Eat Like a Caveman to Achieve a Lean, Strong, Healthy Body.* New York: St. Martin's Paperbacks. ISBN 0312975910.
43. Eaton, S. Boyd; & Konner, Melvin (1985). "Paleolithic nutrition. A consideration of its nature and current implications". *The New England Journal of Medicine* **312** (5): 283–89. PMID 2981409.
44. Taylor, Mike (January 9, 2008). "Refined Food Bad! Caveman Diet Good!", TheStreet.com. Retrieved on January 19, 2008.
45. Eaton, S. Boyd; Shostak, Marjorie; & Konner, Melvin (1988). *The Paleolithic Prescription: A Program of Diet & Exercise and a Design for Living.* New York: Harper & Row. ISBN 0060158719.
46. Sirota, Lorraine Handler; & Greenberg, George (December 1989). "Book reviews". *Applied Psychophysiology and Biofeedback* **14** (4): 347–54. doi:10.1007/BF00999126.
47. Eaton, S. Boyd; Shostak, Marjorie; & Konner, Melvin (1989). *Stone-Age Health Programme.* Angus & Robertson Childrens. ISBN 0207162646.
48. Vines, Gail (August 26, 1989). "Palaeolithic recipe for the clean life / Review of 'The Stone-Age Health Programme' by S. Boyd Eaton, Marjorie Shostak and Melvin Konner", New Scientist. Retrieved on January 19, 2008.
49. Eades, Michael R. & Eades, Mary Dan (2000). *The Protein Power Lifeplan.* New York: Warner Books. ISBN 0446608246.
50. Atkins, Robert C. (1999). *Dr Atkins' New Diet Revolution.* Vermilion. ISBN 0091889480.
51. Worm, Nicolai (2002). *Syndrom X oder ein Mammut auf den Teller. Mit Steinzeit-Diät aus det Wohl stands Falle* (in German). Lünen: Systemed-Verlag. ISBN 3927372234.
52. Cordain, Loren (2002). *The Paleo Diet: Lose Weight and Get Healthy by Eating the Food You Were Designed to Eat.* New York: Wiley. ISBN 0471267554.
53. Cordain, Loren & Friel, Joe (2005). *The Paleo Diet for Athletes: A Nutritional Formula for Peak Athletic Performance.* Rodale Books. ISBN 1594860890.
54. Lindeberg, Staffan (2003). *Maten och folksjukdomarna—ett evolutionsmedicinskt perspektiv* (in Swedish). Lund: Studentlitteratur. ISBN 9144041675.
55. Lindeberg, Staffan. "Home". *Paleolithic Diet in Medical Nutrition.* Retrieved on January 19, 2008.

56. Cordain, Loren. "The Science of Healthy Eating". *The Paleo Diet*. Retrieved on January 19, 2008.
57. Burfoot, Amby (February 11, 2005). "Should you be eating like a Caveman?", Runner's World. Retrieved on January 19, 2008.
58. Shreeve, Jimmy Lee (2007-08-16). "The Stone Age Diet: Why I Eat Like a Caveman", Independent UK. Retrieved on January 19, 2008.
59. Tuttle, Erica (September 4, 2000). "Revolutionary Evolutionary Diets", FindArticles. Retrieved on January 19, 2008.
60. Mysterud, Iver (May 20, 2004). "Kosthold og evolusjon" (in Swedish). *Tidsskr Nor Lægeforen* **124** (10): 1415, http://www.tidsskriftet.no/index.php?vp_SEKS_ID=1021682.
61. Cordain, Loren. "A Sample of Paleo Recipes". *The Paleo Diet*. Retrieved on January 19, 2008.
62. Lindeberg, Staffan. "Frequently Asked Questions: What can I eat?". *Paleolithic Diet in Medical Nutrition*. Retrieved on January 19, 2008.

ABOUT THE AUTHOR

Paul Burke has his Master's Degree in Integrated Studies from Cambridge College in Cambridge, Massachusetts. His life long experience as a champion body

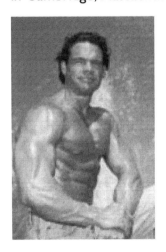

builder, arm wrestler, actor, and an academic professor brought him to write his first book; a very detailed book about exercise, fitness and nutrition for the Mature Male, along with two other written gems about nutrition and weight training that are due for release in June, 2009, and November, 2009 (respectively).

In his first book, "Burke's Law," *A New Fitness Paradigm for the Mature Male*, he makes the very persuasive case for changing the "old fitness training paradigm" to one that he has termed, "Burke's Law," one that incorporates everything from each person finding his own set of "Bio-mechanically perfect exercises," to trying best to eat like his version of our Paleolithic ancestors—elaborated upon in detail in his second book.

Dr. Barry Sears, of 'The Zone" fame, says: "Paul Burke has mastered the understanding that a great body for the mature male is a combination of intelligent training coupled with an equally intelligent diet. Even more impressive is that he has maintained his great physique in the face of a chronic disease that would leave many resigned to a life of inactivity." Almost shocking words, from a historical man in our culture. What makes Burke go on training with a disease that cripples most?

Burke was diagnosed with MS (Multiple Sclerosis) in 1995 while training Bill Koch and his America's Cup Team in San Diego, CA. Says Burke, "How could I," I thought nervously in my head, "the biggest, strongest, most athletic guy who everyone knew as just those things, be headed toward the crippling prospects of Multiple Sclerosis?" "To say the least, my world was turned upside down."

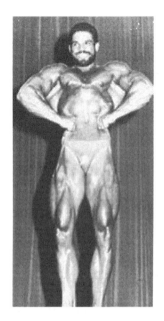

Burke says that MS was the driving force behind his own training paradigm shift and the beginning of a long arduous road back to healing and growing into one of the World's most respected writers and trainers for men over 40. Having been the Over 40 Editor for magazines, "Exercise For Men Only"; "Men's Exercise"; "Natural Body Building & Fitness"; and he is now a monthly columnist for "Iron Man." Between his books and columns, he has developed a large and world-wide following.

Burke's second book, "The Neo-dieter's Handbook," *When We Lost Our Nutritional Roots and Where to Find These Foods Today* (Book-Surge/Amazon, 2009), is being touted by everyone from Dr. Barry Sears to world champion weight trainers and bodybuilders. His third and upcoming book, "Burke's Law II," **Quantified Bodybuilding**: *Reaching Your Muscular Potential Through Musculoskeletal Designation* (Book-Surge/Amazon, 2009) is due to be released this fall. It is the written explanation of how Burke uses his training client's musculoskeletal measurements as a guide to match with bio-mechanically, leverage advantageous exercises—all stored in an enormous database comprised of every possible musculoskeletal measurement, for every human being—with the "proper" exercises for each of those variables.

Many have said that Burke wrote "the wrong book," that the unbelievable story of his life should have been his first published book. Burke started out on his own, very young, and joined the traveling carnival and circus at the age of 16. He had begun lifting weights at the age of 12 years old. Then running the carnival rides, taking them down by hand and traveling over the road with the gigantic machines taught Burke a lot. His curiosity to understand everything from the "strongmen" acts to the movement of the arms on the giant "Spider" ride allowed him to first understand bio-mechanics, machinery and leverage. This led him to join the US Air Force and become a Crew Chief on HH-53 Helicopters, in the *Rescue* branch of the Air Force. It was in the Air Force that Burke won his First Body Building Contest, while stationed in England–the contest, "The Mr. Titian," in London, 1981. Burke soon was honorably discharged from the military, only to move again to the West Coast and train with the big boys: Arnold, Franco, Lou Ferrigno and many other champions. It wasn't long and Burke was winning larger contests and he found himself in New York City, working for Yul Brynner as his body guard at night, while auditioning for his own acting roles during the day. He received his first principal role in a Levi's commercial and received his Screen Actors Guild card in 1983. This led to principal roles in "Spenser For Hire", "Guiding light," and his big break, with Julia Roberts in "Mystic Pizza".

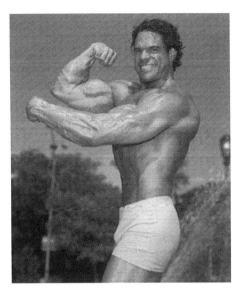

But, something always brought Burke back to Body Building. While living with Franco Rossellini and Doris Duke, on Duke Farms in Somerset, NJ, Burke won the Mr. Empire State Contest and then finished third in both Jr. Mr. USA and Jr. Mr. Universe. Burke's star was on the ascent in many ways, but his love and passion for training with weights always brought him back to wanting more, despite an acting career just waiting for him to grab hold.

Burke began training celebrities and opened his own gym in Cambridge, Massachusetts. The Kendal Athletic Club was in a new building that looked out over a tributary to the Charles River. While gathering clients, Burke introduced himself to the Billionaire son of the richest family in the United States. Bill Koch was at that time just beginning to sail; and Burke offered Koch his training services and as Koch got into shape at Burke's Fitness Club, Koch asked Burke to come and sail with him on the Maxi Boat World Championships and on to the America's Cup. Burke was built to grind the huge mainsail of the Maxi's and soon he was off again to other places, now sailing with Koch in other worldly places.

Eventually, Burke went to work for Koch full time as his trainer and his assistant. It was during Koch's Women's Team trial for the Cup that Burke began getting symptoms of MS.

"Bill (Koch), sent me to his house on Oyster Harbors to recover, but it took me years to get better." Not long after, Burke was on his own, lying in bed wondering what life would bring him. He started researching diet from an evolution standpoint and he wondered if all of his years of heavy, day after day type training hadn't contributed somehow to his health problems.

Finally, Burke recovered and began training a different way, eating differently and soon his body looked better than ever. "Burke's Law" was born and off to New York City he went to do more acting and training. To this day Burke contends that in every miserable experience there is some kind of silver lining. "I would have never written this book if I didn't get MS, and rupture my assessor nerve," he says as if he planned it that way. True, his life was full of travel and adventure and his

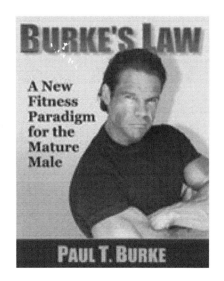

BURKE'S LAW

A New Fitness Paradigm for the Mature Male

PAUL T. BURKE

admirers are many; yet, Burke always goes back to where he began. "I began lifting weights and marveling at the workings of the Human Body, and I suppose that is where my passion will always remain." "Burke's Law" is a book like no other. To quote Steve Cardillo, the inventor of the Reebok "Pump" Belt and National Power lifting Champion, "Paul Burke never ceases to amaze me—he is simply the most talented genius I have ever met."

This book, "Paul Burke's Neo-Dieter's Handbook," *When We Lost Our Nutritional Roots; Where to Find Those Foods Today* is another gem of Burke's flexing his ability to weave almost poetic like verbiage, combining his experiential wisdom with his empirical knowledge— within two subject genres that are usually dull and tediously cookie-cutter boring. His approach is always the same whether writing about Nutrition, Body Building, Fitness, or specifically detailed questions posed to him from readers of his monthly column in "Iron Man" magazine (the country's oldest "Iron" Magazine): He has "eagle" eyes and a "mouse" type ability to cull the greatest of detail and still see the world from afar. This book will leave you feeling as if there is no other "human diet" possible than the one he puts forth. No tricks, no magic bullet and no smoke and mirrors. It is Burke's interpretation of history telling us all what the future of "dieting" is.

For more information about Burke's books, go to www.Amazon.com

Go to Paul's website: www.paulburkefitness.com

"Burke's Law," (Trafford Publishing, 2006, Amazon Book-Surge Publishing, 2009).

"Paul Burke's Neo-Dieter's Handbook," *When We Lost Our Nutritional Roots; Where to Find These Foods Today.* (Amazon Book-Surge Publishing, 2009).

This book is a Book-Surge/Amazon, Paul Burke Enterprises, LLC collaboration.

Made in the USA
Lexington, KY
26 January 2013